Palgrave Studies in Risk, Crime and Society

Series Editors

Kieran McCartan, Department of Criminology, University of the West of England, Bristol, UK
Beth Weaver, School of Social Work and Social Policy, University of Strathclyde, Glasgow, UK

Risk is a major contemporary issue which has widespread implications for theory, policy, governance, public protection, professional practice and societal understandings of crime and criminal justice. The potential harm associated with risk can lead to uncertainty, fear and conflict as well as disproportionate, ineffective and ill-judged state responses to perceived risk and risky groups. Risk, Crime and Society is a series featuring monographs and edited collections which examine the notion of risk, the risky behaviour of individuals and groups, as well as state responses to risk and its consequences in contemporary society. The series will include critical examinations of the notion of risk and the problematic nature of state responses to perceived risk. While Risk, Crime and Society will consider the problems associated with 'mainstream' risky groups including sex offenders, terrorists and white collar criminals, it welcomes scholarly analysis which broadens our understanding of how risk is defined, interpreted and managed. Risk, Crime and Society examines risk in contemporary society through the multi-disciplinary perspectives of law, criminology and socio-legal studies and will feature work that is theoretical as well as empirical in nature.

Kieran McCartan · Anne Eason ·
Sarah Senker · Nick Addis · Cody Porter
Editors

Developing and Implementing a Public Health and Criminological Approach to Tackling Sexual Abuse

Prevention, Treatment and Integration

palgrave
macmillan

Editors
Kieran McCartan
University of the West of England
Bristol, UK

Anne Eason
University of the West of England
Bristol, UK

Sarah Senker
University of the West of England
Bristol, UK

Nick Addis
University of the West of England
Bristol, UK

Cody Porter
University of the West of England
Bristol, UK

ISSN 2946-2517 ISSN 2946-2525 (electronic)
Palgrave Studies in Risk, Crime and Society
ISBN 978-3-031-93633-3 ISBN 978-3-031-93634-0 (eBook)
https://doi.org/10.1007/978-3-031-93634-0

Cover illustration: SEAN GLADWELL/Gettyimages

This Palgrave Macmillan imprint is published by the registered company Springer Nature Switzerland AG
The registered company address is: Gewerbestrasse 11, 6330 Cham, Switzerland

Foreword

This book represents the power of collaboration and synergy, where different concepts combine to create something greater than their individual parts. The complexities of child sexual abuse and sexual violence demand such a multifaceted approach as no single perspective can encompass the breadth of these issues. It is through the integration of varied insights, spanning disciplines, experiences, and approaches that we unlock innovation, foster creativity, and illuminate pathways towards effective solutions to complex problems.

In 2022, I received a Churchill Fellowship to explore the need for a public health framework to address child sexual abuse in the UK. This fellowship allowed me to travel to North America for several months, where I met with experts in child sexual abuse prevention and treatment. Highlights included presenting the widely adopted UK Harmful Sexual Behaviour framework at the Association for the Treatment and Prevention of Sexual Abuse (ATSA) 2022 conference in Los Angeles, spending a week in residence with the Department of Human Development and Family Studies at Pennsylvania State University, and sharing ideas and challenges with colleagues at the Johns Hopkins Bloomberg School of

Public Health in Baltimore. There was a strong consensus among all I spoke with that adopting a public health approach to sexual abuse prevention has great potential as a framework to organise, structure and develop our thinking.

Historically, prevention programs in both the United States and the UK have often lacked a theoretical basis. Many were shaped by outdated and inaccurate perceptions of abusers—for instance, the overemphasis on 'stranger danger'—and placed disproportionate responsibility on children and young people to protect themselves, rather than fostering collective accountability across society. Numerous experts in the United States have acknowledged that primary prevention efforts have predominantly focused on teaching personal safety skills to school-aged children, with the aim of equipping them to prevent victimisation.

However, it is crucial to reiterate that the onus of preventing sexual abuse does not lie with the child. Abuse arises not from a child's vulnerability, but from an offender's inclination and ability to exploit that vulnerability. Recognising this is essential to refocusing prevention efforts on systemic and societal solutions that address the root causes of abuse.

Integrating criminal justice theory with public health approaches offers a promising pathway for developing the practical steps urgently needed to address sexual violence and abuse. An effective public health model must account for the dynamic interplay between individual vulnerabilities or dispositions and situational factors in shaping human behaviour. This nuanced understanding is essential for identifying the conditions that contribute to sexually abusive behaviour and for crafting targeted interventions. Whilst these concepts remain relatively new to the field of sexual violence and abuse, contributions such as this book, highlight the role that Epidemiological Criminology (EpiCrim) prevention techniques can play in advancing prevention efforts and fostering meaningful progress in this area.

Together for Childhood—Community Specific Prevention

We have a real opportunity to understand and explore what it really looks like to prevent child sexual abuse in a community through the place-based initiatives that are currently running in several locations in the UK. 'Together for Childhood' is an ambitious 10-year place-based partnership approach to prevention originally designed by the NSPCC, seeking to understand and address problems at a local level in a truly integrated way, with a focus on community capacity-building and evidence-based development. The ambition is to deliver a programme that goes beyond simply developing several evidence-based services to support children and families, but instead, to create a wide-reaching project that creates sustainable systems change and engages local people to get involved in thinking about and understanding how they can contribute to keeping children safe within their community.

This book strongly advocates for Epidemiological Criminology (EpiCrim) approaches to the prevention of sexual abuse, emphasising interventions across multiple population levels—individual, interpersonal, community, and societal—and at various stages of offending, including before, during, and after incidents occur. The Together for Childhood initiative exemplifies these principles of the Epi Crim approach. It employs a theory of change grounded in public health philosophy to identify gaps, commission interventions, and develop activities. Like EpiCrim, it is deeply rooted in the social and behavioural ecosystems of specific communities, viewing child sexual abuse as a community issue with far-reaching individual impacts. This perspective underscores the importance of a collective, community-based response to addressing such abuse.

Emerging research and evaluations reveal encouraging trends, demonstrating that better community understanding of child abuse fosters improved relationships and cooperation between the public, communities, and professional stakeholders, such as those in health, justice, education, and charitable sectors. Significantly, these efforts have also led to increased reporting of abuse. However, this local progress contrasts sharply with the current direction of UK national data in 2025, where statistics indicate a concerning 8% decline in the identification of sexual harm compared to the previous year (CSA Centre of expertise on child sexual abuse, 2025).

Amidst these challenges, there remains hope. Professor Jennie Noll, Director of Mount Hope Family Centre in New York, has recently published groundbreaking data demonstrating that coordinated, community-wide primary prevention initiatives can reduce both substantiated and unsubstantiated cases of child sexual abuse at the population level. Her innovative use of synthetic control methods and insightful comparisons with prior statewide policies provide compelling evidence of the transformative potential of such efforts. In stark contrast to ongoing legislation that has failed to protect children, her findings offer a powerful and instructive model for meaningful progress.

A Role for All

The very implications of a public health approach mean an effective preventative response will require effort from all areas of society—at individual, relational, family, community, societal and system levels. This is important and translates to mean that every child, parent/carer, teacher, social worker, healthcare professional who works with children, family member, and friend should understand what child sexual abuse is and know how they can play a part in preventing it. Which leads us to the importance of the message.

We need to be clear how communities and the public in general are currently framing and understanding sexual abuse and violence because this can help focus and refine prevention messaging and the type of discourse and conversations that are likely to gain best traction. Whilst not all professionals or sectors of society are yet able to fully conceptualise the idea of public health methodology, there is much more unity and support for the principles of the prevention of harm and abuse underpinning a public health approach. Wider engagement and collaboration will come from the framing of child sexual abuse as a preventable public health problem and strengthening societal resolve that child sexual abuse can be prevented. This kind of public outreach serves various purposes, not the least of which is acknowledging the serious problem of child sexual abuse publicly, communicating to both (potential) offenders and victims, that they are not alone in this experience, and encourage access to services. The more we encourage public awareness of the problem, the more we can anticipate behavioural change, even if only by suggestion (e.g. increased monitoring, supervision).

Why isn't more being done in the UK to prevent child sexual abuse before it happens?

This book is part of the response and solution as it underscores the need to address child sexual abuse as a public health issue employing more than a singular framework. It promotes a comprehensive understanding enabling the integration of existing frameworks and theoretical models to design effective interventions and prevention strategies. The solution, therefore, lies in the interplay of theoretical foundations and the collaboration of professionals to construct a cohesive and multidisciplinary framework—one that is accessible for all disciplines.

Significant progress is now underway to establish a widely adopted and accessible public health-informed national prevention framework to tackle child sexual abuse in the UK. Grounded in valuable lessons from prevention initiatives across the UK, the United States, and internationally, this framework is being developed to serve as a vital resource for local authorities, safeguarding partnerships, and central government departments. It aims to shape both local and national policies and practices, ensuring that preventative strategies are prioritised in the funding of future activities and initiatives. Now we must examine how this emerging framework can effectively integrate and amplify ideas from EpiCrim, reaffirming the principle that 'the whole is indeed greater than the sum of its parts'.

London, UK
March 2025

Pat Branigan
Assistant Director, NSPCC

Pat Branigan is the associate head of Development at the NSPCC and leads the charity's response to child sexual abuse with a focus on preventing harmful sexual behaviour displayed by children and young people. In addition to this, he's an anthropologist with a background in public health and has led research into sensitive sexual health topics at the London School of Hygiene & Tropical Medicine.

Contents

Notes on Contributors

Nick Addis, PhD, is a senior lecturer in Criminology at the University of the West of England (UWE), UK, where he teaches modules on criminal/forensic psychology, research methods, and crime prevention. He is currently involved in a series of projects focusing on the prevention of sexual violence across different settings, and, together with colleagues, has established the Preventing Sexual Violence seminar series over the 2022/23 academic year. Before joining UWE Bristol, Nick was employed as a senior lecturer in criminology at Sheffield Hallam University, where he was the course leader for the BSc (Hons.) Criminology and Psychology degree. Nick has over 10 years' experience teaching in higher education, and has teaching experience across a number of areas, including the fields of criminological theory, criminal justice, offender rehabilitation, mental health, risk assessment, sexual offending, study skills, research methods, geographical information systems/spatial analysis, and policing and crime reduction.

Geraldine Akerman is a forensic psychologist who has worked in prisons with men who have committed sexual and other violent offences for 25 years employed by HMPPS and more recently by the NHS. She has published papers and presented at national and international conferences on the subjects of Therapeutic Communities, sexual offending, compassion-focused therapy, mental health in prison, and transitioning through custody many co-authored by those in custody. Geraldine is a visiting lecturer at the University of Birmingham, where she was awarded her PhD, and at Cardiff Metropolitan University, where she was awarded the Honorary Professor role. Geraldine is the Deputy Chair of the Division of Forensic Psychology.

Helen Bovill, PhD, is an associate professor at the University of the West of England (UWE), Bristol, in the College of Health, Science and Society and the School of Education and Childhood. Helen's research interests include Relationships, Health and Sex Education Provision within schools, and prevention of gender-based violence within education and society, Helen has been involved in work exploring bystander awareness and intervention to prevent and respond to VAWG in a university setting. Helen has been interviewing students from Police and Education and related allied professions, and their lecturers to understand more about supporting these students to become ambassadors against VAWG. Helen is also currently researching provision for relationship and sex education within schools with an aim of preventing and responding to VAWG in an earlier phase. Helen predominantly teaches/supervises postgraduates at UWE and is Director of Studies for a range of edd and PhD students. Helen is an editorial board member for the 'Journal of International Women's Studies' and is a member of the Review Panel for Research Papers in Education alongside peer reviewing for 'Journal of Sexual Aggression', 'Widening Participation and Lifelong Learning', 'International Journal of Lifelong Education', and 'British Educational Research Journal'.

Maggie Brennan, PhD, is an assistant professor in Psychology at Dublin City University. Maggie has worked on research and policy initiatives to combat Online Child Sexual Exploitation and Abuse (OCSEA) for over 20 years. Her work includes multi-disciplinary collaborations with major domain stakeholders such as NGOs (e.g. National Centre for Missing and Exploited Children), law enforcement agencies (e.g. Interpol), cross-government forums (e.g. G7 countries) and social media companies.

Maggie is a co-founder of cybersafekids and the International Working Group for the Prevention of Online Sex Offending (IWG_OSO). Maggie is also a Fellow of the Higher Education Academy. She teaches on a range of undergraduate and postgraduate programmes in DCU, including the 'DCU Futures' Psychology of Disruptive Technologies and Psychology and Mathematics programmes.

Lol Burke, PhD, is Professor in Criminal Justice at Liverpool John Moore's University and specialises in the areas of probation research, policy and practice. He has an extensive publication record in CJ/Probation. These include co-authored monographs 'Delivering Rehabilitation' (Routledge 2014) and 'Redemption, Rehabilitation and Risk Management' (Routledge 2011), chapters in 7 edited collections, and over thirty published outputs in refereed journals and professional publications. He has an outstanding record of research and external income generation, being part of a team that secured a major ESRC grant (2014) and a European Commission award (2012). He has nationally/internationally recognised external engagement activities and achievements across a wide range of professional and governmental bodies, including especially: NAPO, The Howard League, and Probation Institute. Lol has impressive links with probation work in Europe, has represented NAPO at an event in the House of Lords, provided evidence to the Justice Committee, and has given keynote speeches across Europe and to the American Society of Criminology. He was editor of the leading Probation Journal from 2007–2016 and is on the editorial board of the European Journal of Probation. He is a Fellow of the HE.

Phil Cawley is the lead restorative justice trainer for Lancashire Constabulary and in addition to being a restorative justice practitioner, his role is to promote restorative justice across Lancashire Police and with other agencies and partners. He is currently undertaking a PhD at Liverpool John Moores University. His research investigates why more men convicted of a sexual offence do not engage with restorative justice. Phil is also a membership trustee of the Restorative Justice Council.

Anne Eason, dcrimj, is an associate head of Dept. (Policing) at the University of the West of England, UK, overseeing the Police Constable

Degree Apprenticeship. She is also a Trustee of The Wheels Project, Bristol, and a charitable organisation that provides alternative education for young people who need support in the development of vocational and social capital. A former Senior Probation Officer, her operational expertise is in the field of risk assessment and management of high risk of harm offenders and her research interests are in domestic abuse and violent offences against women and girls, emotional intelligence and decision-making in police education. Recent research focuses on trauma informed practices with sexual offenders and children's perception of police and racial discrimination. Dr Eason has a growing number of publications, most recently *A Police Officers Guide to Academic Research*, Palgrave Macmillan.

Paul Gavin, PhD, is a senior lecturer in Criminology in the School of Social Sciences at the University of the West of England (UWE) Bristol. He is a former graduate of University of Galway, Kings College London and holds a doctorate in Criminology from Kingston University London. His research interests include restorative justice, problem solving justice and mental health. He has previously worked as a researcher with the National Commission on Restorative Justice and the National Crime Council in Dublin and with the Centre for Crime and Justice Studies in London.

Elizabeth Green, MSc, main research interests are around the management of data access and applications of microdata in decision-making. Her current research explores the application of European data management model—'5 safes' in different cultural contexts. She holds a future data services fellowship award for the ESRC working with the Future Data Services (FDS) programme which aims to establish the next generation of data services.

Ian Johnson is currently Associate Head of Department/Cluster Leader for Cyber Security & Business Computing within the department of Computer Science & Creative Technology. He is responsible for leading around 27 staff. Prior to this he was AHOD Information Science, and before that programme leader for the B.Sc. Forensic Computing & Security programme (now renamed Cyber security & Digital Forensics). He is Co-Director of our Gold recognised NCSC Academic Centre of Excellence in Cyber Security Education, one of only 7 in UK. He is a highly experienced teacher and academic with a history of programme and module design. He has designed and led modules for nearly thirty years in a number of programmes from the MSc Parallel Computer Systems (1989) through the MSc Systems Administration and Security, to the current undergraduate Forensic Computing & Security programme for which he led the redesign in 2016. His main interests are networks & network security, operating systems and embedded systems and he has previously led modules in these areas. He has interests covering a wide gamut of cyber security issues, from embedded systems security, through network forensics to the tracability of digital currency transactions.

Emily Jones Chartered Forensic Psychologist, St. Andrews Healthcare. Emily Jones is a forensic psychologist who trained at HMP Grendon, working with men who have committed sexual and other violent offences. More recently Emily has joined St. Andrews Healthcare and is working in the Learning Disability and Autism division. She has published papers on the subjects of Psychologist wellbeing during the COVID-19 pandemic, Therapeutic communities and more recently on sexual offending.

Hazel Kemshall is currently Emeritus Professor of Community and Criminal Justice at De Montfort University. She has research interests in risk assessment and management of offenders, effective work in multi-agency public protection, and implementing effective practice with high-risk offenders. She has completed research for the Economic and Social Research Council, the Home Office, Ministry of Justice, the Scottish Government, the Risk Management Authority, and the European Union. She has over 150 publications on risk. She has completed research into European information exchange systems on serious violent and sexual offenders who travel across EU borders and produced training manuals for Police, Prisons and Probation across Europe. Working with a range of agencies she has also developed organisational and practice responses to combatting violence against women across all EU Member States. She is a leading expert in Multi-Agency Public Protection Panels and the management of high-risk offenders in the community, risk assessment, and combining risk and desistance approaches to offender management. She has researched the facilitation of self-disclosure by sexual offenders (moj), public awareness campaigns for combating sexual offending (Leverhulme), and reintegration of high-risk offenders into the community including the use of Circles of Support and Accountability (moj). She recently assisted Her Majesty's Prison and Probation Service to complete the risk of harm guidance for prison and probation staff in England and Wales.

Stephanie Kewley, PhD, is a professor of Forensic and Criminal Justice and is currently seconded to the Centre of expertise on child sexual abuse as Principal Research and Evaluation Officer. Stephanie has worked for the last two decades in Criminal Justice and Forensic Psychology research, educational, and correctional contexts. The central focus of her work is the prevention of sexual violence, in particular, how secondary prevention strategies might help prevent sexual abuse from occurring in the first place. Stephanie's work aims to support, advocate and promote, the safe and healthy functioning of marginalised and highly stigmatised populations involved and/or incarcerated by criminal justice structures and systems. Her research engages peoples unique lived experience as well as the professionals who support them. Stephanie works across multi-disciplinary research, policy and practitioner teams, and her research portfolio examines aspects of vulnerability, risk and need in the context of sexual violence prevention, offender rehabilitation, risk management, public protection, child protection, criminal and social justice, public health, and prisoner human rights.

The UK research infrastructure for academics working with confidential data is largely based on his work. She is a Senior Strategic Fellow for the ESRC Future Data Services programme, and regularly provides formal and informal advice on data governance and data access to government, academia and health services. His work has been a major influence across the world, leading directly to primary legislation in the UK and Australia. He is an active researcher, with a focus on the disadvantaged in society. Although specialising in the quantitative analysis of confidential secondary data, he regularly works with colleagues on qualitative and mixed-methods collecting primary data

Sophie King-Hill, PhD, is an associate professor in the Health Services Management Centre at the University of Birmingham, UK. She specialises in sexual behaviours and assessment in children and young people, sexual health, sibling sexual behaviour/abuse, misogyny, relationships & sex education and the importance of youth voice. Much of her work is cross-sector, cross-disciplinary and centred around participatory and stakeholder co-design approaches. Sophie also has an interest in policy implementation, transfer and success frameworks and evaluation strategies. Previously she worked extensively in the third sector in the field of education and sexual health with many diverse groups such as teenage parents and young people with social, emotional and behavioural difficulties.

Phil Legg, PhD, is a full professor in Cyber Security effective from January 2022. I am Co-Director of the uwecyber Academic Centre of Excellence in Cyber Security Education (ACE-CSE), as recognised by the National Cyber Security Centre (NCSC), and I am Programme Leader for the NCSC-certified MSc Cyber Security. His research interests address the intersections of cyber security, machine learning, visual analytics, and human-computer interaction, including improving interpretability and understanding of risk, and improving robustness and trust of modern security technologies. Previous research has addressed insider threat detection and cyber situational awareness, through to human-machine teaming for assessing confidence and trust of multiple agents, and active adversarial machine learning for identifying security vulnerabilities in dynamic learning systems.

Kieran McCartan, PhD, is a professor of Criminology at the University of the West of England (UK). He has a track record of public, academic and professional engagement on criminological issues, including the origins and causes of sex offending, and societal responses to sex offenders. He has developed a wide-ranging, multi-disciplinary network around sex offender management and reintegration. He has experience of qualitative, quantitative and mixed method research from funders including Ministry of Justice, Cabinet Office, Public Health England, ESRC, The Leverhulme Trust, Bristol City Council & Wiltshire probation. Professor McCartan is currently the Deputy Chair of National

Organization for the Treatment of Abuse, a member of the Confederation of European Probation working group on sexual offences, a member of the ethics committee of Brave hearts and is a member of the International Working Group for the Prevention of Online Sex Offending. Professor mccartan has advised the Council of Europe, New Zealand Police, Bravehearts as well as Department of the Prime Minister and Cabinet, Australia.

Hannah Merdian, PhD, is an associate professor and the Deputy Head of the School of Psychology, Sport Science and Wellbeing at the University of Lincoln. She is co-director of onlinePROTECT®, a research and consultation programme on online child protection. She has published widely on the needs and risks of individuals who have accessed child sexual exploitation material and has worked with a range of charities, partner organisations and treatment providers to support evidence-based decision-making. Her child protection research presented a highly rated impact case study in the UK's 2021 Research Excellence Framework.

Jane Meyrick, PhD, is dual qualified as Chartered Health Psychologist (registered HCPC) and a Public Health Specialist (Fellow of the Faculty of Public Health). She teaches across the Health Psychology post graduate portfolio on the evidence base and sexual health/violence. She brings the key elements of her professional backgrounds (lived experience and wider prevalence/determinants) to her research work at UWE Bristol on marginalised communities in sexual health including survivors of sexual violence. She is an active member of the Psychological Sciences Research Group. She has worked in front line services, central policy making and research across public health and sexual health for over 25 years and recently published an accessible, evidence-based overview of sexual violence and harassment with a focus on what works to prevent, the work aims to help inform the building of safer communities, #metoo for Women and Men.

Chris Pawson, PhD, is a psychologist and researcher working in the field of mental health and wellbeing. Specifically, he applies participatory methods and community psychological frameworks in research and promotion of mental health among those experiencing multiple exclusion through homelessness, domestic abuse and addiction. Chris previously worked with the U.K. Home Office evaluating interventions for young people and their families and working with youth offending teams and in prisons. Chris is currently evaluating interventions funded by the National Health Service and U.K. Government in the South West of England.

Cody Porter, PhD, is Senior Lecturer and Psychology Programme Lead in the School of Social Sciences at the University of the West of England (UWE) Bristol. She completed her PhD Psychology at the University of Portsmouth and worked in the NHS previously supporting patients with wellness and recovery. She has published various research articles within the field of Forensic Psychology and has consulted with several organisations. Her research primarily focuses upon investigative interview, lie-detection and offender employability, and she is the Deputy Journal Editor for the Investigative Interviewing Research & Practice journal.

David S. Prescott is a mental health practitioner of 39 years, David Prescott is the Director of the Safer Society Continuing Education Center. In that capacity he has overseen more than 90 live online CE trainings and 80 webinars with a combined total of 37,000 participants. Mr. Prescott is the author and editor of 25 books in the areas of understanding and improving services to at-risk clients. Mr. Prescott is best known for his work in the areas of understanding, assessing, and treating sexual violence and trauma, including with adolescents and young adults. Mr. Prescott is the recipient of the 2014 Distinguished Contribution Award from the Association for the Treatment and Prevention of Sexual Abuse (ATSA), the 2018 recipient of the National Adolescent Perpetration Network's C. Henry Kempe Lifetime Achievement award, and the 2022 recipient of the Fay Honey Knopp Award from the New York State Alliance for the Prevention of Sexual Abuse and New York State ATSA. He also served as ATSA President in 2008–09. Mr. Prescott currently trains and lectures around the world. His published work has been translated into Japanese, Korean, German, French, Polish, Dutch, and other languages. He has served on the editorial boards of four scholarly journals. He has been the co-author of the monthly NEARI and MASOC newsletters since 2007, which are read by several thousand professionals who work with adolescents who have sexually abused. Since 2011, he has served as Co-Blogger for ATSA's Sexual Abuse blog, which has been read over 850,000 times and was recently rated among the top blogs in the world on the topic

Ella Rees, MSc, is a research associate at the University of West of England (UWE), Bristol, working in the School of Social Sciences and School of Education and Childhood in the College of Health, Science and Society. Ella is currently involved in a range of projects relating to the prevention of sexual violence and child sexual exploitation within her role in Social Sciences (Criminology) as well as supporting a variety of projects within Education, as well as the Education and Childhood Research Group (ECRG). She has previously worked in the field of child sexual exploitation prevention as well as alongside the criminal justice system. Ella has research interests in male violence against women and girls, restorative justice and practice and trauma informed practice.

Felix Ritchie is a leader in the governance of confidential data for research purposes. He conceived the 'Five Safes', the dominant governance framework for social science data in the public sector and academia. He and his colleagues have created new philosophies of data governance, and practical tools such as output checking guidelines. With Elizabeth Green, he has developed best-practice training for researchers and research data managers. In 2022 Green and Ritchie were commissioned by the National Institute for Health Research to provide data governance training for four years across their whole portfolio of research projects in low- and middle-income countries.

Sarah Senker, PhD, is a research associate at the University of the West of England (UK) and visiting fellow at the University of Royal Holloway, supervising students on the MSc Forensic Psychology. As a chartered psychologist and published author, Sarah has worked as an independent research consultant since 2011 undertaking projects for the Ministry of Justice, Independent Inquiry into Child Sexual Abuse, Home Office and NHS England. Sarah has undertaken work in over 55 prisons in England and Wales and specialises in qualitative research methods. Her particular research interests are in the rehabilitation of people with sexual convictions, the application of trauma informed approaches and preventing domestic abuse. She has presented on her research findings at both a national and international level.

Nadia Wager, PhD, is a professor in Psychology at Teesside University. She has a long history of evaluating community interventions for victims of serious crimes whilst working in partnership with those delivering the services. Her primary areas of research interest are; measuring the extent, impact, prevention, and societal responses to victimisation, particularly in relation to sexual victimisation and modern slavery.

List of Figures

List of Tables

1

Preface

Kieran McCartan, Anne Eason, Sarah Senker, Nick Addis, and Cody Porter

Introduction

This book is based on a body of research stretching over the past 15 years at the University of the West of England, Bristol (UWE, Bristol) on public health approaches to sexual abuse. The book focuses on work by internal and external colleagues to the university on a range of sexually abusive behaviours and interventions as well as how they have implemented into policy and practice locally, nationally and internationally. The edited collection is a collection of chapters that define the area of EpiCrim and then given research, policy and practice insights into how UWE, and related research had driven the field forward. In this introduction we will spell out the context in which this research took place, outlet the research areas, discussed the conference that this work fed into and how the book highlights and builds on this work.

K. McCartan (✉) · A. Eason · S. Senker · N. Addis · C. Porter
University of the Westestest of England, Bristol, United Kingdom
e-mail: kieran.mccartan@uwe.ac.uk

K. McCartan et al. (eds.), *Developing and Implementing a Public Health and Criminological Approach to Tackling Sexual Abuse*, Palgrave Studies in Risk, Crime and Society, https://doi.org/10.1007/978-3-031-93634-0_1

Public Health Approaches to Sexual Abuse: UWE Context

UWE Bristol has a strong research history in the social sciences, especially in criminology, psychology and public health that places a place based, city wide, approach at the heart of its research and practice. The city region of Bristol is often a testing ground for staff across the university to research and apply ideas, interventions, and policies in a real world setting. Bristol is a large, multi-culturally regional capital and therefore has a diverse population, socio-economic landscape and several population-based challenges (including, health, justice, and education) which makes it an ideal place to examine at and understand complex social issues like sexual abuse. Much of the preliminary work of this collection, and the related research, is based on the work of Professor Kieran McCartan who has sought to understand the roots causes of sexual abuse, especially child sexual abuse, and how to best prevent first time as well as repeat offending (McCartan et al., 2018; McCartan et al., 2020; Bovill et al., 2020; McCartan et al., 2021; McCartan et al., 2023; Kemshall & Mccartan, 2022; McCartan, and Kemshall, 2020; McCartan et al., 2020; McCartan, 2022).

In doing research in the area of the prevention of sexual abuse an Epidemiological Criminology (EpiCrim) approach was used and adapted, based on the intinal work of Lanier (2010), over many years and publications by McCartan (McCartan et al., 2023; Kemshall and Mccartan, 2022; McCartan and Kemshall, 2020; McCartan et al., 2020; McCartan, 2022). An EpiCrim approach to understanding, preventing and responding to sexual abuse states that you need to intervene at different population levels (*individual, interpersonal, community, and societal*) and at different points in the offending trajectory, pre/early offending (*primary and secondary prevention*) and post offending (*tertiary and quandary prevention*) through working with people at risk of being a victim of and/or someone who will cause sexual harm, to stop it from happening. This is rooted in an evidenced base, multidisciplinary, systematic approach (*for a further discussion of the EpiCrim framework and how it ties to preventing and responding to sexual abuse see chapter 2*) (Fig. 1.1).

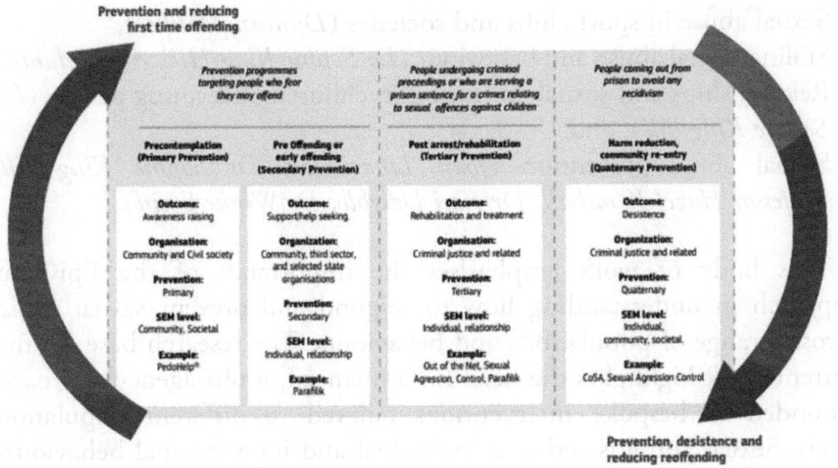

Fig. 1.1 Public health approach to the prevention of Child sexual abuse (Di Gioia et al., 2022)

Professor McCartan has collaborated with several internal and external colleagues, as well as external organisations (National Organisation for the Treatment of Abuse, Association for the Treatment and prevention of Sexual abuse, NSPCC, Barnardo's, Lucy Faithful Foundation, Circles UK, Circles South West, Confederation of Europe Probation, The European Union and European commission) on a range of projects including,

- Risk and risk management (*Professor Hazel Kemshall, Dr Anne Eason, Dr Cody Porter*)
- Online sexual offending and child sexual abuse material (*Dr Nick Addis, Dr Hannah Meridian, Dr Maggie Brennan*)
- Community integration of people convicted of a sexual offence (*Professor Kelly Richards, Dr Robin Wilson, Professor Hazel Kemshall*)
- Trauma informed practice (*Dr Anne Eason, Professor Hazel Kemshall, Dr Chris Pawson, Dr Sarah Senker*)
- Campus based sexual abuse prevention and campus climate surveys (*Dr Jane Meyrick, Professor Phil Rumney, Dr Nick Addis, Dr Helen Bovill, Professor Rachel Fenton, Aga Kowalska*),

- Sexual abuse in sport clubs and societies (*Duncan McPhee*),
- Sibling sexual abuse and behaviour (*Dr Sophie King-Hill, Amy Adams*),
- Relationships and sexual education in children and young people (*Dr Sophie King hill*), and
- Sexual abuse prevention (*Joan Tabachnick, Dr Sophie King-Hill, Professor Hazel Kemshall, Dr Kasi Uzieblo, Dr Winke Smid*).

This body of work emphasises the importance of the EpiCrim approach in understanding how to respond and prevent sexual abuse across a range of populations and behaviours. The research base for the current book highlights the need for a nuanced, multi-agency approach grounded in bespoke interventions tailored to different population levels. Sexual abuse is series of individual and interpersonal behaviours influenced by community and societal values and beliefs therefore responding to and preventing sexual abuse needs to be responsive to populational and social needs, as well as those of individuals.

In 2020 there was an opportunity to apply for internal research funding at UWE to develop research clusters around emerging areas of excellence. A research team, led by McCartan, submitted a proposal to develop a cluster related to EpiCrim approaches to preventing and responding to sexual abuse. This work proposed the development of a larger internal and external multi-disciplinary research network to bring together expertise from criminology, psychology, sociology, policing, public health, education and cybercrime to work on the prevention of sexual abuse. The internal application was funded, and the network was established.

- **Internal academic members**: Professor Kieran McCartan, Dr Anne Eason, Dr. Nick Addis, Dr. Helen Bovill, Dr. Paul Gavin, Dr Finn MacKay, Charlotte Kite, Duncan McPhee, Dr Jane Meyrick, Dr Chris Pawson, Dr Amber Phillips, Dr Cody Porter, Ella Rees, Dr Sarah Senker, Dr Zoe Thomas, Professor Philip Legg, Ian Johnstone.
- **External academic members**: Professor Hazel Kemshall, Dr. Sophie King-Hill, Professor Sarah Brown, Professor Geri Ackerman, Dr Maggie Brennan, Professor Kelly Richards, & Amy Adams.

– **Partner organisations**: European Commission, Circles Southwest, Nation Organization for the Treatment of Abuse, NSPCC, Together for Childhood, Bristol North Somerset & Soth Gloucestershire integrated care board, Avon & Somerset police, His Majesty's Prison & Probation Service, Thriving Survivors, HMP Grendon, HMP Leyhill, Office of the Regional Director of Public Health Southwest NHS England, SARSAS/Rape crisis.

The research network recruited three research associates (Dr Sarah Senker, Ella Rees, & Charlotte Pritchard) and set about conducting real-world research. The cluster is structured around four research and practice areas (1) Community & societal understanding of sexual abuse (primary prevention), (2) Working with "at risk" populations (secondary prevention); (30 Treatment & rehabilitation (tertiary prevention); & (4) Harm reduction, desistence, and integration (quaternary prevention). It focused on two streams of work,

1. Helping communities to understand and engage with sexual abuse to assist "at risk" populations

   This area of work bridges areas of work, (1) Community & societal understanding of sexual abuse (primary prevention) & (2) working with "at risk" populations (secondary prevention). This area of research focuses on research, policy development, and knowledge exchange examining primary and secondary prevention with victims as well as people who are at risk of committing sexual abuse. This area stream of work examined how best to prevent sexual abuse in communities. In this area, most of the research and practice revolves around messaging, bystander intervention, and media narratives. This research looked to examine the issue at a place based, community level as most of the research and practice to date focuses on individual actions and behaviours. It focused on communities in Bristol (including, geographical communities, social communities, and professional communities) looking at how these communities come together (or don't) to understand and respond to victims as well as people who commit sexual abuse; particularly in terms of actual offending being observed in situ or responding to post disclosure. The research examined how in individuals get their information and how they use that, or don't use that, to support, develop, or intervene in the community. In doing this research, we can build more bespoke and fit for purpose knowledge and support for communities so that they can prevent, intervene, and engage in community integration for both people who have been a victim as well as a preparator of sexual abuse. In doing so, the research wanted to understand how best to move the framing of sexual abuse intervention, prevention, and engagement with those impacted from a "responsibility" (which indicates choice) to "expectation" (which indicates requirement), and some of the best practice in this area.

2. Supporting recovery from sexual abuse in both victims and "perpetrators"

   This area of research, policy development, and knowledge exchange work focused on harm reduction, desistence, and integration (quaternary prevention). This area work looked at innovate ways to integrate people impacted in sexual abuse, both victims and people convicted of a sexual abuse, back into the community post offence. For victims this would be about facilitating their recovery and for individuals convicted of a sexual offence this would be about the process of desistance, harm reduction, and effective risk management. The area used recovery capital to frame these debates, but practically the emerging idea of justice capital and how it links to quaternary prevention (i.e. do no harm). The research examined professional, policy maker and service user perspectives on this and how we can build a clear framework for developing a harm reduction and restorative process. In addition, the research looked at incorporate strengths-based approaches, restorative justice, community support, employer support, innovations around low-level offenders and rehabilitative culture.

Over the following 18 months the research cluster developed and carried out research oin these two areas, resulting in publications, further funding and impact. At the same time McCartan with Rachel Campbell (Health & Justice Lead Southwest, NHS England) and Helen Erswell (Public Health Wales) set up thew Public Health and Criminal Justice Southwest Network. The network was established as a mechanism to bring a broad range of professionals and academics together from across the Southwest to discuss issues relating to criminal, justice, health and public health. The network current has approximately 300 members and runs a series of in personal, hybrid and online events. One of these events was the "Developing professional and policy understandings of the role of EpiCrim in preventing and responding to sexual abuse" conference in June 2024.

EpiCrim Conference 2024

The conference was a one-day event to showcase the research that was taking place at UWE on EpiCrim approaches to understanding, preventing and responding to sexual abuse. The presentations were all part of the research network with some being internal and external to the university. The event was attended by over 100 partners, collaborators and professionals from across the UK that worked in the field of sexual abuse. The conference was split into four sections, after a general introduction to the day and EpiCrim from McCartan, these were.

1. **Prevention**
    a. Examining the role of online communities in the prevention of child sexual abuse - Dr Nick Addis, Ella Rees, Ian Johnson, Professor Phil Legg, & Dr Maggie Brennan
    b. Building an Informed workforce to prevent and respond to VAWG - Dr Helen Bovill and Ella Rees
    c. Understanding disclosure of sexual violence/abuse across different settings and points of intervention - Dr Jane Meyrick
2. **Treatment**
    a. Issues, Challenges, and Opportunities for Trauma Informed Practice - Dr Sarah Senker, Dr Anne Eason, Dr Chris Pawson
    b. Developing a trauma informed work force: the role of compassion in treatment and rehabilitation - Professor Geri Akerman, HMP Grendon, & Emily Jones, HMP Grendon

   c. Keeping practitioners safe: Looking after the health and wellbeing of the professional and compassion fatigue - Dr Anne Eason

3. **Integration**

   a. Restorative Justice as a response to sexual violence Dr Paul Gavin, Dr Cody Porter, & Dr Phil Cawley, Liverpool John Moore's University
   b. Employability barriers for those with a sexual conviction - Dr Cody Porter & Dr Hannah Merdian, University of Lincoln
   c. Circles of Support and Accountability: An EpiCrim approach rooted in restorative practice - Professor Kieran McCartan, Professor Kelly Richards, QUT Brisbane, & Dr Robin Wilson, Wilson Associates

4. **KPI'S and evaluation**

   a. Developing a solid research base, methodology and data sets for EpiCrim - Professor Felix Richie & Elizabeth Green,
   b. Developing KPI and evaluation criteria in practice: Sibling Sexual Behaviour/Abuse - David Russell, Thriving Survivors, & Amy Addams, University of Birmingham.

Across the event there was great professional, academic and practice engagement highlighting the many challenges and opportunities that the prevention of sexual abuses posed and how an EpiCrim approach might work to help resolve these. The main discussion points and outcomes from the conference were captured in an infographic (Fig. 1.2) which highlighted the importance of multi-agency working in a community centred, child focused approach to prevention of sexual abuse. The conference highlighted that it is essential to place community understandings and useable, practical approaches at the centre of any preventable approach to sexual abuse.

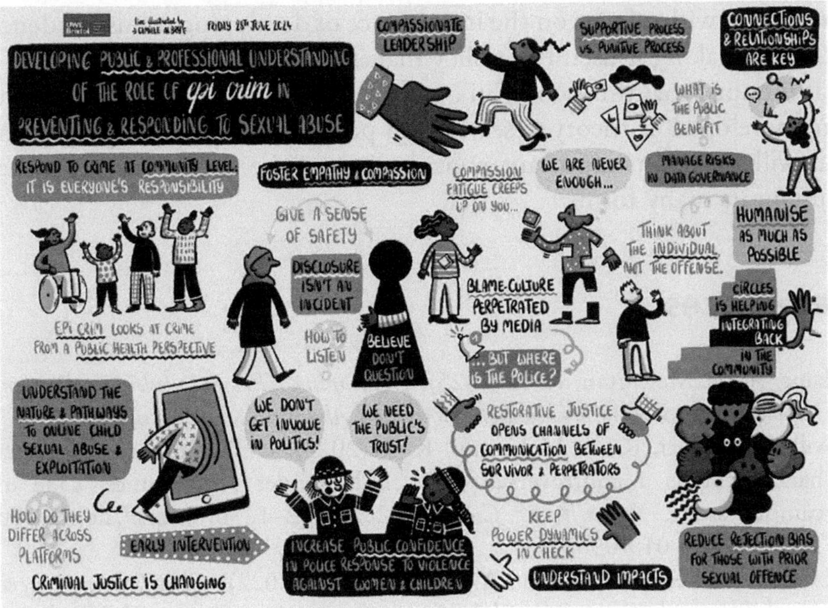

Fig. 1.2 Infographic on the use of an EpiCrim framework to prevent and respond to sexual abuse

The Development, Structure and Content of the EpiCrim Book

The current book follows the structure of the conference and leans into the research presented at it as well as the implications for policy and practice. The book omits two areas of research presented at the conference, the paper on sibling sexual behaviour—abuse as that is published elsewhere (Adams & McCartan, 2025) and the paper on Circles of Support and Accountability as a form for EpiCrim practice as that has been published previously (Kemshall & Mccartan, 2022); both are the subjects of ongoing research. The book adds a chapter on multi-agency working within an EpiCrim framework by Hazel Kemshall and a chapter on treatment by David Prescott as it was felt that these where import issues omitted from the conference. The book, like the conference, is structured around the themes of prevention, treatment and community integration with a focus on the importance of developing robust evidence base and making it useful to policy makers and practitioners.

It is hoped that this book will be an important addition to the continuing developed of theory, research and practice in the field og Epic rim and will make an important contribution to the prevention of sexual abuse in its many forms.

References

Adams, A., & McCartan, K. F. (2025). *Developing KPI's for understanding and responding to Sibling Sexual Behaviour and Abuse*. UWE Bristol.

Bovill, H., Waller, R., & McCartan, K. F. (2020). Discussing atypical sexual harassment as a controversial issue in bystander programmes: One uk campus study. *Sexuality & Culture., 24*, 1252–1270. https://doi.org/10.1007/s12119-019-09682-8

Di Gioia, R., Besley, L., Cassar, A., & Pawula, A. (2022). *Classification criteria for child sexual abuse and exploitation prevention programmes*. JRC Technical Report. European Commission.

Kemshall, H., & McCartan, K. F. (2022). *Desistance, recovery, and justice capital: Putting it all together*. HM Inspectorate of Probation.

Lainer, M. M. (2010). Epidemiological criminology (EpiCrim): Definition and application. *Journal of Theoretical and Philosophical Criminology, 2*(1), 63–103.

McCartan, K. F., Merdian, H., Perkins, D., & Kettlebrough, D. (2018). The ethics of secondary prevention approaches with individuals at risk of committing sexual harm. *International Journal of Offender Therapy and Comparative Criminology., 62*(9), 2548–2566. https://doi.org/10.1177/0306624X17723951

McCartan, K. F. (2022). *Adapting out thinking on theory and practice in working with people convicted of a sexual offence*. HM Inspectorate of Probation. HM Inspectorate of Probation.

McCartan, K., & Kemshall, H. (2020). The potential role of recovery capital in stopping sexual offending: Lessons from circles of support and accountability to enrich practice. *Irish Probation Journal, 17*, 87–106. http://www.probation.ie/EN/PB/0/1B01C0821143FED68025862C005298DC/$File/Kieran%20McCartan%20and%20Hazel%20Kemshall.pdf

McCartan, K. F., & Richards, K. (2020). The integration of people convicted of a sexual offence into the community and their (risk) management. *Current Psychiatric Reports., 23*, 52. https://doi.org/10.1007/s11920-021-01258-4

McCartan, K. F., Harris, D. A., & Prescott, D. (2021). “Seen and not heard”: Understanding the service user voice in sex offending treatment & (re)intergration. *International Journal Offender Therapy Comparative Criminology., 65*(12), 1299–1315. https://doi.org/10.1177/0306624X19851671

McCartan, K., & Kemshall, H. (2020). The potential role of recovery capital in stopping sexual offending: Lessons from circles of support and accountability to enrich practice. *Irish Probation Journal, 17*, 87–106. http://www.probation.ie/EN/PB/0/1B01C0821143FED68025862C005298DC/$File/Kieran%20McCartan%20and%20Hazel%20Kemshall.pdf

McCartan, K., & Kemshall, H. (2023). Incorporating quaternary prevention: Understanding the full scope of public health practices in sexual abuse prevention. *International Journal of Offender Therapy and Comparative Criminology, 67*(2–3), 224–246. https://doi.org/10.1177/0306624X211049204

McCartan, K., Uzieblo, K., & Smid, W. J. (2020). (2021). Professionals' understandings of and attitudes to the prevention of sexual abuse: An international exploratory study. *International Journal of Offender Therapy and Comparative Criminology, 65*(8), 815–831. https://doi.org/10.1177/0306624X20919706

Part I

Concept, Context and Evaluation Frames

2

Understating the Epidemiological Criminology Approach and How It Relates to Preventing Sexual Abuse

Kieran McCartan and Sophie King-Hill

Introduction

Sexual abuse and exploitation are local, national, international, and transnational issues that impact people of all races, genders and cultures. Sexual abuse is a significant global issue made more challenging by the fact that there is a significant social and political focus on responding to reported cases of sexual abuse as opposed to other forms of criminal behaviours. The current approach to sexual abuse is rooted in criminal justice the criminal justice system, which means they are focused on supporting victim recovery, seeking justice for the victim, holding the person who has committed the sexual abuse accountability, and seeking to successfully integrate them into society (Uzieblo et al., 2022). Currently there is more focus on the recovery from sexual abuse rather

K. McCartan (✉)
University of the West of England, Bristol, UK

S. King-Hill
University of Birmingham, Birmingham, UK

K. McCartan et al. (eds.), *Developing and Implementing a Public Health and Criminological Approach to Tackling Sexual Abuse*, Palgrave Studies in Risk, Crime and Society, https://doi.org/10.1007/978-3-031-93634-0_2

than the prevention of it. Sexual abuse includes an array of online and offline, contact and non-contact offences that occur within and across borders which means that it's a complex range of offences and behaviours and, therefore, needs a nuanced, multi-faceted shared response (Proulx et al., 2020). The challenge of understanding the scale and nature of sexual abuse, apart from its varying offence types, is that it is typically under reported with victims often not officially disclosing to the authorities and seeking help and/or justice (Meyrick et al., 2024). Although, reporting rates have improved in recent years with societal shifts around the way that we understand and perceive sexual abuse (Meyrick, 2022), current figures still do not reflect the reality of sexual abuse nationally or globally (Childlight, 2025).

Over the last 30 years considerations have emerged as to whether sexual abuse, especially child sexual abuse, can be prevented from happening and not just responded to (Smallbone et al, 2008; Brown, 2017; Kemshall, 2017; King-Hill, 2022a). The sexual abuse prevention policy and practice conversation, especially in respect to CSA, was strongly argued for as part of the childhood matters inquiry in 1997 (King-Hill, 2022a). Initially the prevention of sexual abuse was theoretical, and any studies or practices were small scale resulting in difficulty for policy makers to engage with, but there is now a distinct shift due to the socio-political landscape locally, nationally and transnationally (Merdian et al., 2019; Gioia & Beslay, 2023; Di Gioia, Besley, Cassar, & Pawula, 2022). There is recognition that sexual abuse is preventable through the adoption of an Epidemiological Criminology (EpiCrim) perspective (Kemshall & McCartan, 2022; Lainer, 2010). This chapter will discuss the changing landscape of our response to sexual abuse, but particularly child sexual abuse/exploitation (CSA), focusing on why prevention has become central to current approaches, and what this means moving forward.

The Nature of Sexual Abuse and the Scale of the Problem

The challenge presented by sexual abuse is that it is a broad spectrum of behaviours, actions, and offences. Sexually abusive behaviour is rooted in discussions around mental health, psychological illness, paraphilias, neurodiversity, anti-social behaviours, and exploitation (Proulx et al, 2020). It is important to state that sexual abuse can have a lot of motivating factors not all of which are sexual (Toates et al., 2017). Sexual abuse can be tied to behaviours motivated by domestic violence, hate crime, gang activity, exploitation, bullying for example, and it is essential to understand the motivating factor behind the sexual abuse so that it can be responded to in the most effective way. Therefore, the sexual abuse act that takes place may be being used as a method of harm rather than solely for sexual gratification. Sexual abuse also can involve a lot of different actors, adults and children, each with their own underlying motivations and vulnerabilities. The reality is that when we talk about sexual abuse it is important to consider that it is not a single heterogeneous concept, rather a range of behaviours committed by one individual (or a group of individuals) against another within or across their age group, gender, nationality, or culture. This is amplified when thinking about sexual abuse transnationally and across cultures, as a not everyone characterises sexual abuse in the same way and the law is not universal with different countries having different offences and prosecution thresholds (ECPAT International, 2024). For this chapter, when referring to children and young people this will include those under the age of 18 as set out by the United Nations Rights of the Child (UNRC) (United Nations, 2022).

When thinking about how to prevent and respond to sexual abuse exploration of the population in question needs to take place, looking at the aspects that pertain the broader societal and community factors as well as their individual factors. In recognising that sexual abuse is complex, it needs a range of approaches as well as a variety of public, professional and policy engagement to enable us to build a holistic approach (McCartan, 2022). Therefore, all forms of sexually abuse behaviour and offences need to be considered equally. For instance, when CSA is discussed, there needs to be recognition that a significant proportion of it is peer-on-peer (harmful sexual behaviour in children and young people—HSB-CYP) and therefore need to consider how children and young people at risk are engaged with (King-Hill, 2023, 2024; King-Hill & McCartan, 2024). Building comprehensive engagement models around sexual abuse is the best way of making sure that the appropriate prevention messaging is sent and received (Prevention Global, 2025). Additionally, this approach reinforces the important of an EpiCrim approach and then need to move away from traditional messaging.

The exact figures for the range and scale of sexual abuse in general or (as named behaviours or offences) is unknown, which means that understanding the true extent of the abuse, as well as its impacts, is challenging (Dworkin et al., 2021). Which means that understanding, predicting and responding to sexual abuse is problematic and complex. It is important to recognise that different organisations, agencies and disciplines use different overarching language, some talk about Gender Based Violence (GBV), or violence against women and girls (VAWG), or sexual abuse (SA) as all-encompassing terms, which can be political and problematic. The reality is that the focus on violence against women and children (VAWC) in the context of sexual abuse as this represents the reality of most of the harm. In this chapter we will us the organisations own terminology in reporting their data.

The United Nations (UN) states that one in three people (736 million) have been a victim of physical and/or sexual intimate partner violence, non-partner sexual violence, or both at least once in their life (30 per cent of women aged 15 and older). However, most violence is committed by current or former intimate partners with more than 640 million women aged 15 and older (26 per cent) have been subjected to intimate partner violence (UN, 2024). When the prevalence of sexual abuse is examined, the UN indicates that 6% of women report they have been subjected to sexual violence from someone other than their husband or partner, and approximately 15 million adolescent girls worldwide, aged 15–19 years, have experienced rape. Research indicates that although sexual abuse exists in every country worldwide, it disproportionately affects low- and lower-middle-income countries and regions, with 37% of women aged 15 to 49 living in countries classified by the Sustainable Development Goals as "least developed" have been subject to physical and/or sexual intimate partner violence in their life. The true prevalence of non-partner sexual violence is likely to be much higher, considering the stigma related to this form of violence. The exact figures for the prevalence of CSA globally is not known, as its under reported and under recorded, a UNICEF report cites figures that state that 1 in 8 of the world's children (12.7%) had been sexually abused before reaching the age of 18 (UNICEF, 2020). we are This points to it being a silent epidemic, Research indicates that CSA is a global issue that existing in every country internationally (UNICEF, 2021; United Nations, 2014, 2020), and that it is a growing issue. In the UK research by the Centre for expertise in Child Sexual Abuse (CSA Centre) indicates that one in 10 children in England and Wales are sexually abused before the age of 16, however this is thought to be an underestimate given low-reporting and recording rates, as well as issues linked to official recording practices and agency data..

However, this is an ongoing issue and not just linked to CSA but also to all sexual offences, including rape (Victim Commissioner, 2021) with system level issues impacting reporting, recording and prosecutions and falsely shifting social perception of the prevalence and reality of sexual abuse.

To understand sexual abuse, comprehension of the full range of behaviours and interactions is needed, which means understanding the reality and impact of HSB-CYP, because as well as a form of peer-on-peer abuse it is also a form of CSA. Research and evidence indicate that most HSB-CYP is committed by CYP known to each other and in relationships (HMI Probation, 2025). The evidence suggests that in England and Wales nearly half of young people aged between 13 and 17 who have been in a relationship in the past year have experienced violent or controlling behaviour, with over half of the 106,984 child sexual abuse cases reported in 2022 involving young people aged between10 and 17 (King-Hill & McCartan, 2024). In addition, there is an emerging research base that indicates that sibling sexual behaviour-abuse (SSB-A) is more prominent in nature than originally assumed and is one of the most common forms of intra-familial violence and abuse (King-Hill et al., 2023; King-Hill and McCartan, 2024).

In respect to online sexual abuse, the UN indicates that the prevalence of online violence gender-based violence (OGBV) ranges from 16 to 58%, with Facebook as the top location (see chapter 3 for more discussion of the role of online platforms) (Hicks, 2021). Individuals who commit online sexual abuse and CSA report divergent, multi-faceted and often over-lapping motivations for their actions, which has been highlighted in recent research by protect children on child sexual abuse material (CSAM) users (please see the EU Horizon 2020 funded projects PROTECT CHILDREN, 2025, and PROTECH, 2025) and evidence from the #metoo movement (Meyrick, 2022). Current research by Childlight states that in the last 12 months 300 million plus children were affected by CSA, 1 in 8 where subjected to online grooming and where exposed to non-consensual taking and sharing of online sexual material, and that one case of abuse is reported every second (Child light, 2024). Research indicates that the underlying drivers of online sexual abuse and harassment centre around power and control, with a focus on heteronormative expectations around gender roles and sexual practice. It is important that violent and sexually abusive behaviours are understood on a continuum as not all behaviours are as abusive and problematic as each other, although the impact that they have on the victim can be significant regardless. This is currently observed in HSB-CYP (Hackett continuum, Hackett, 2010; brook traffic light tool, Brooke, 2025) but these are not without their practice limitations (King-Hill, 2022b). However, this is not generally carried out with adults in respect to sexual abusive behaviours. Therefore, we need to consider the continuum of sexual behaviours and abuse for adults upon adults in the online and offline spaces, keeping in mind that the crossover between online and offline sexual behaviours is not always straight forward, direct or easily understood (Brennan et al., 2019).

Research indicates that the financial cost of violence against women and girls, including but not limited to sexual abuse, is significant across the EU-27 at more than EUR 290 billion (European Union, 2021). However, this cost is a likely underestimate as violence against women and girls is a complex problem that can affect the lives of the victims, those close to them and society, both directly and indirectly, making it particularly difficult to capture the full extent of the effects of violence in costing studies. Also, if violence against women and *children* is considered, so including all genders of those under 18, the cost will increase significantly and be more representative of the reality of sexual abuse across society.

Despite the under-recording and low-reporting nature, more cases of sexual abuse are discovered, reported, and recorded annually (UN, 2025). It is important to note that with changing community and societal attitudes to sexual abuse, especially CSA, improved and more evidence-based policing as well as an increased drive for more prosecutions we are seeing an increase in the reported prevalence of sexual abuse, though this maybe a false positive with the actual rates only really being fully understood. Therefore, we might not be seeing an increase in sexual abuse but rather have a better understanding of the actual rates of sexual abuse in society.

Additionally, with the ever-changing nature of sexual abuse including the mediums through which it happens (*the increase in online sexual abuse*), the role of technology (*the rapid development of AI generated CSAM*), and the introduction of new categories of sexual abuse (*sibling sexual behaviour and abuse*) our understanding of the scale and nature of sexual abuse is ever changing. Research, policy and practice guidelines from a range of national and transnational organisations including, CSA Centre, End Child Prostitution in Asian Tourism (ECPAT INTERNATIONAL), Internet Watch Foundation (IWF), WE Protect Global Alliance who all highlight and reference this and it has started to feed into the way that we respond to and prevent sexual abuse locally, nationally, and transnationally (Di Gioia et al., in press). Therefore, there needs to be consistent reviewing of approaches in responding to and preventing sexual abuse in the light of an expanding evidence base, always being critical and reflective of past approaches and interventions.

The Need for a Different Approach in the Changing Landscape of Criminal Justice

Traditionally sexual abuse is seen as a criminal justice and policing issue (McCartan, 2022), with the role of the state to respond to reported cases of sexual abuse; however, based on research, policy, and practice over the last 30 years this approach does not seem to be reducing the scale and nature of sexual abuse (Brown, 2017; McCartan & Gotch, 2020; King-Hill, 2022a).). Research highlights that sexual abuse has the lowest recidivism rates of all forms of violence, and that with the correct pro-social interventions risk from this population can, and will, reduce over time (McCartan & Gotch, 2022). However, criminal justice interventions alone cannot achieve this. Most offences are committed by people unknown to the police (Wilson, Sandler & McCartan, 2020), which means focusing the attention at reducing re-offending, although important, would not prevent or reduce most sexual abuse from occurring (Tabachnick, & Klein, 2011). To realistically reduce sexual abuse, in all its forms, changes and approach are needed and the role of the state requires consideration (Di Gioia et al, 2022; McCartan, 2022). One of the ways that this can be achieved is through looking to prevent, not just respond to, sexual abuse.

The prevention of sexual abuse sits within a larger crime prevention movement which focuses on stopping criminogenic behaviour before it happens, therefore resulting in no victim, and therefore no cost, to the criminal justice system, and an increases community safety (Sutton et al., 2021; Wager et al., 2021; Ellefsen et al., 2023).

One of the main theoretical models that underpins most crime prevention initiatives outlines four key strategies: (1) education, (2) risk mitigation, (3) risk management, and (4) direct action (Ellefsen et al., 2023). Therefore, crime prevention occurs by educating individuals and communities about the impact and consequences of criminogenic behaviour, putting in place barriers and deterrents that make committing crime harder as well as taking direct actions with riskier or more challenging populations. The logic of crime prevention works with all forms of criminogenic behaviour, including but not limited to sexual abuse. Preventing sexual abuse is about educating individuals and communities, putting in place social sanctions that make sexual abuse more difficult and support individuals to seek help and not offend. While there has been progress over the years (Prevention Global, 2025) with the prevention of sexual abuse starting to be recognised as being a key policy and practice platform for all major international organisations and intergovernmental organisations (i.e., the United Nations, European Union, World Health Organisation), there is still more to do at the national and local level with government and professional bodies having to realign, develop and implement these perspectives.

The proliferation in crime prevention strategies that have been developed have not always translated to increased, or improved, sexual abuse prevention, especially with at risk communities. Harris et al. (2024) states that this has been carried out in an inconsistent and "haphazard" fashion. Consequentially, there has been an active move in policy and practice to reframe sexual abuse, especially CSA, as a health and wellbeing issue over the last 30 years within the academic and practice spheres with a recognition that health and wellbeing issues directly and indirectly contribute to the preparation of sexual abuse and are a consequence of it (Brown, 2017; Kemshall, 2017; King-Hill, 2022a). This fits in with a growing recognition by policy makers and government that criminogenic behaviour is underpinned key criminological and psychological theories of the causes of crime, including, life-course analyses of offending behaviour, trauma, adverse childhood experiences (ACE's), rehabilitation, and desistence (Kemshall & McCartan, 2022; McCartan & Kemshall, 2023; McGee & Farrington, 2019). This highlights the importance of multidisciplinary work in criminal justice, and that by doing so it opens opportunities for innovation and collaboration in crime reduction, community safety and risk management than traditional, punitive models. A public health is approach looks to reduce the causes of poor health and wellbeing across different population levels and cohorts through a range of different, targeted interventions (NHS, 2025). In respect to sexual abuse, this means reducing the causes of offending behaviour, improving the health and wellbeing of people at risk of committing a sexual offence as well as those directly, and indirectly, effected by it. The idea behind public health is that different populations need different types and styles of interventions and that these should be evidence based and fit for purpose. With the recognition that criminogenic behaviour is a health and wellbeing issue, this means that a public health approach can be developed and used (Kemshall & McCartan, 2022).

Epidemiological Criminology

Epidemiological Criminology (EpiCrim) (Lainer, 2010) is the theoretical and academic framework that the prevention of sexual abuse is situated. EpiCrim is a recognition that the fields of criminology and health need to work together to allow understanding of the causes and consequences of offending behaviour better (Lainer, 2010).

> *This is the explicit merging of epidemiological and criminal justice theory, methods, and practice. Consequently, it draws from both criminology and public health for its epistemological foundation. As such, EpiCrim involves the study of anything that affects the health of a society, be it: crime, flu epidemics, global warming, human trafficking, substance abuse, terrorism or HIV/AIDS.* (Lainer, 2010, p. 72).

EpiCrim views sexual abuse as a behaviour, like other social behaviours, rather than an event. Typically, from a criminal justice perspective we focus on the index offence (i.e., the offence that the person was arrested and convicted off) rather than the array of behaviours and actions that lead up and surrounded that behaviour. It sets out that sexual abuse can be prevented through interventions at different points in the criminogenic trajectory. An EpiCrim approach argues that crime and offending behaviours are a form of social interaction which is rooted in the nature/nurture debate and reflects the bio-psycho-social model of developmental criminology, rehabilitation, desistance, trauma informed practice currently used within the criminal justice system (see: Bradley, 2017; Pringer & Wagner, 2020; McGee & Farrington, 2019; McCartan, 2022; McCartan & Kemshall, 2023). Taking an EpiCrim approach recognises the multi-disciplinary nature of criminal justice practice (see Chapter 3 in this book) and reinforces that the most effective response to crime requires individualised as well and large-scale, contextual explanations to develop appropriate interventions. An EpiCrim approach reinforces a growing recognition that sexual offending, including CSA, is a community, developmental, and life-course issue (Brown, 2017; Kemshall, 2017; McCartan et al., 2015a, 2015b, 2021; NSPCC, 2024), which enables proactive response focused on communities, and risky populations as well as individuals, utilising prevention strategies rooted in health education and knowledge application (McCartan, Kemshall, & Tabachnick, 2015a; NSPCC, 2024) (see Fig. 2.1 for an infographic laying out the different aspects of sexual abuse within a EpiCrim frame).

The EpiCrim approach explains prevention across two axes; the socio-ecological model and the preventive stages. Both of which are underpin understanding the EpiCri approach and how it relates to the role of law enforcement in preventing and responding to sexual abuse.

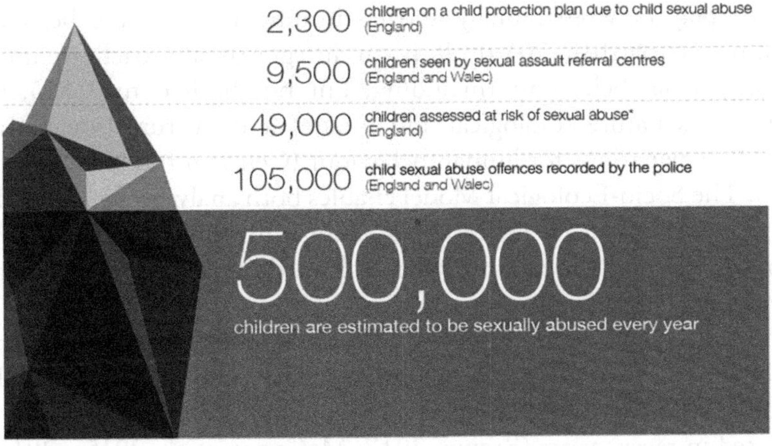

Fig. 2.1 The scale of child sexual abuse compared with agencies' identification of it

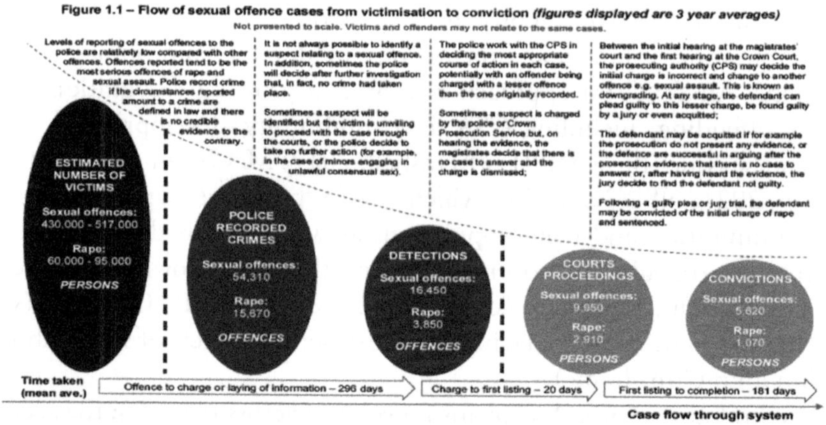

Fig. 2.2 Flow of sexual offences cases from victimisation to conviction (ONS,.nd)

Social Ecological Model

The first axis of the EpiCrim approach is a population based, or a person/place-based approach that requires consideration of how different groups are engaged with and how this reduces the risk of offending. The Socio-Ecological Model (SEM) is positioned as central to the EpiCrim approach as it essentially devises prevention strategies as it emphasises the interplay between biology and environment in shaping behaviour (Colding & Barthel, 2019). It is an integrated approach to understanding social behaviour (including, but not limited to, CSA), that incorporates nature (biological and innate) and nurture (societal and learned) explanations for human behaviour (Centre for Disease Control, 2004). The Socio-Ecological Model enables both analysis of and an effective response to, social issues by targeting different population levels, including the individual, interpersonal/relationship, community, and societal (see Fig. 2.3).

The SEM has been applied to both non-sexual crimes (Fisher-Kowalski, 2015), and sexual offending (Smallbone et al., 2008). The use of SEM in understanding and responding to sexual offending has increased in recent years (Brown, 2017; McCartan et al., 2015a, 2015b), as its "tiered" system allows other disciplines to clearly see how they

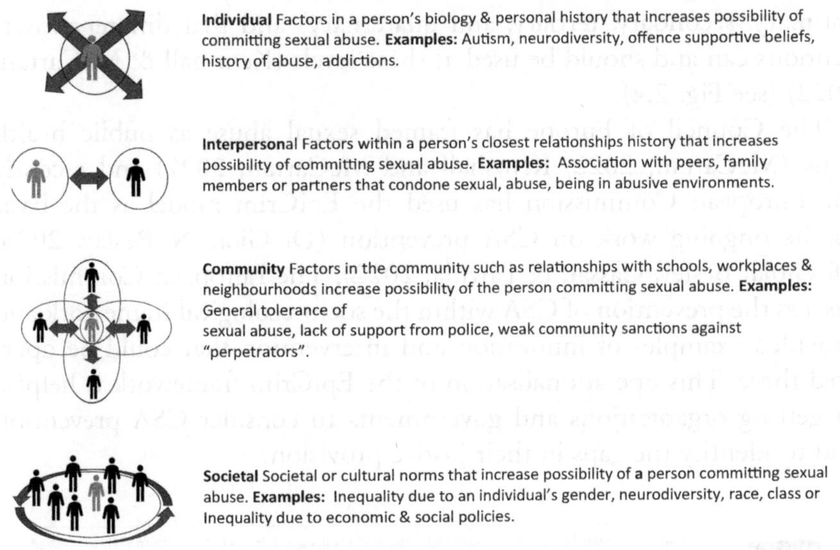

Fig. 2.3 The socio-ecological model preventing and responding to sexual abuse

fit into the prevention and response to sexual abuse. Public health approaches in sexual abuse have drawn heavily on SEM, particularly in terms of research and advocacy for more effective responses (see: Brown, 2017; Kemshall & Moulden, 2017; Letourneau et al., 2014).

Prevention Stages

The second axis of the EpiCrim model focuses on the point and the time of intervention in correspondence to the criminogenic behaviour; addressing the prevention of first-time offending as well as reducing re-offending. An EpiCrim approach is a harm reduction model, which makes sense in health and public health, but at times struggles in criminal justice because of the nature, structure, and responsibilities of criminal justice organisations, especially law enforcement (Senker et al, 2023). An EpiCrim approach argues that there are four levels of prevention (primary, secondary, tertiary, and quaternary) and that different interventions can and should be used at these levels (Kemshall & McCartan, 2022) (see Fig. 2.4).

The Council of Europe has framed sexual abuse as public health issue (McCartan, 2022; Kemshall and McCartan, 2022) and recently the European Commission has used the EpiCrim model as the basis for its ongoing work on CSA prevention (Di Gioia & Beslay, 2023; Di Gioia, Besley, Cassar, & Pawula, 2022). The European Commission discuss the prevention of CSA within the socio-ecological framework and provided examples of innovation and intervention that could be operated there. This operationalisation of the EpiCrim framework is helpful in getting organisations and governments to consider CSA prevention and to identify the gaps in their justice provision.

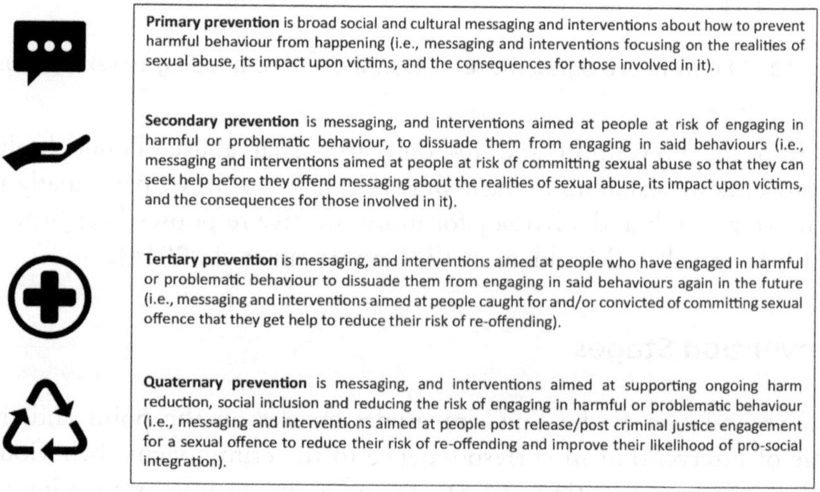

Fig. 2.4 The four prevention stages

EpiCrim: Practice, Framing, and Engagement with Sexual Abuse

The idea that sexual abuse is preventable is well established (Smallbone et al, 2008; Brown, 2017; Kemshall, 2017) there is a clear rationale for why this should happen (Tabachnick & Klien, 2011; Di Gioia et al, 2022), with work having been done to consider how this is framed at a public, policy, and practice level (McCartan, Kemshall, & Tabachnick, 2015a, 2015b). However, the framing and the messaging around sexual abuse prevention is an important step in creating understanding of this issue with a range of populations. If populations across wider society do not understand it or see how it relates to them, their actions, and/or their lives they will not engage (Prevention Global, 2025; NSPCC, 2025). The challenge of messaging around sexual abuse, especially sexual abuse prevention, is that it is confounded by perpetrator and victim myths, social disengagement, and moral positioning of the subject area, as well as a lack of nuanced and realistic media/political messaging around this (Global Prevention, 2025; Kitzinger, 2004). Conversations in the sexual abuse field are tied to debates on imprisonment, punishment, and victims' rights which can make debates about prevention, especially prevention focusing on men who have harmed or are about to harm difficult (Letourneau, 2024). The social perspective is punitive and focussed upon exclusion rather than being focussed on rehabilitation and inclusion. There is a different conversation about this sexual abuse population compared to other offending populations (i.e., fraud and anti-social behaviour) and other public health crisis (i.e., smoking and cancer), which makes it more challenging to have a nuanced debate (Letourneau, 2024).

It is important to recognise that these social norms and socio-cultural beliefs on sexual abuse are rooted in experiences, systems, culture, personality and behaviours making them both personal and societal, therefore they can bc difficult to change (Banyard et al., 2020). In the past 30 years since the childhood matters inquiry (King-Hill, 2022a) there has been a focus on developing increased population knowledge about sexual abuse (i.e., rape, child sexual abuse and online sexual abuse/exploitation) through changes in government policy and messaging, campaigns by charities and Non-Government Organisations (NGO's), media engagement and debate (including, but not limited to the use of soap operas, documentaries) which has resulted in sexual abuse having a higher socio-political profile (Independent Inquiry into Child Sexual Abuse, 2022; King-Hill, 2022a). However, although there has been an increase in social awareness of sexual abuse, and sexual abuse prevention, this does not necessarily mean that social views and values around this have changed (Independent Inquiry into Child Sexual Abuse, 2022). Recent research by John Hopkins (Global Prevention, 2025) as part of the global prevention initiative indicates that the two most common narratives used by the public in the framing of CSA is:

(1) **The Law and Punishment Narrative** which is post offence and the person who commits CSA is seen as unimaginably "bad" and/or being so mentally unwell that they inevitably commit abuse, while the survivor is portrayed as being forever damaged.
(2) **The Vigilant Child Narrative** which is preventing CSA through individual action and responsibility. This narrative tells a story that individual children (and their caregivers to some extent) need to be constantly vigilant for signs of potential predators in their midst and that they are solely responsible for preventing abuse.

As a result of their research Prevention Global developed and tested a new public/community narrative to understand CSA prevention—**the help provided narrative** (Prevention Global, 2025). This framing of CSA prevention focuses on problematic systems that do not work to prevent child sexual abuse, therefore lifting the narrative from the individual and interrelationship levels to that of the community and society (as outlined in Fig. 2.3 & 2.5). This states that child sexual abuse is a community issue and therefore different communities (or systems) need to work together more effective to reduce the climate where individual can engage in sexually harmful behaviour and to strengthen interpersonal connections between people so that they can seek help and better understand child sexual abuse.

Which mirrors CSA prevention work and messaging being carried out in the UK currently. For example, the NSPCC have a particular

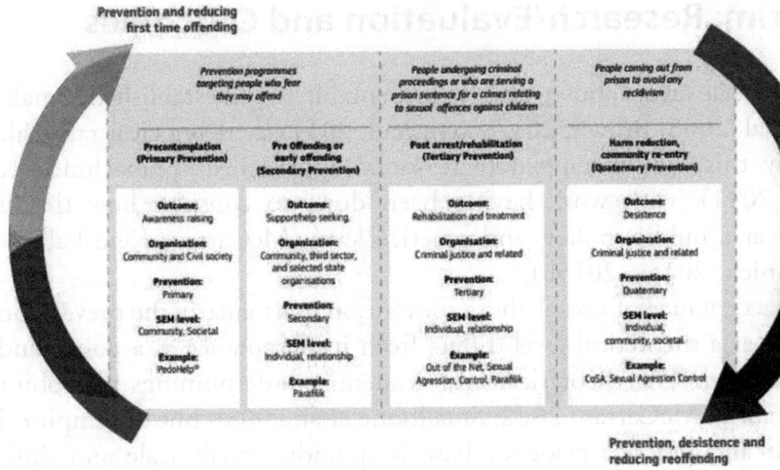

Fig. 2.5 Prevention initiatives within the prevention stages (Gioia & Beslay, 2023)

focus on this through current work that they are doing in communities through Together for Childhood (TFC) a place-based approach to the prevention of child sexual abuse, abuse, and neglect (NSPCC, 2025). The initial research indicates that TFC has increased community awareness of a range of child sexual abuse and that they feel empowered to work with professionals to increase prevention activities. Although these examples are focusing on contact child sexual abuse in the main, there are related projects looking at online child sexual abuse (Protect children - 2KNOW, 2025), working with men at risk of committing child sexual abuse (Prevent to protect - 2PS), supporting frontline professionals to engage better with communities around child sexual abuse (ECPAT International) as well as broader forms of sexual abuse including rape (Rape Crisis). With changing social, cultural and political narratives around sexual abuse and argument that sexual abuse can be prevented and framed as a public health, health and wellbeing issuc there needs to be a robust evaluation frame to allow is to monitor as well as evaluate this change.

EpiCrim: Research/Evaluation and Outcomes

The idea that sexual abuse, CSA, is preventable is well established (Smallbone et al, 2008; Brown, 2017; Kemshall, 2017) there is a clear rationale for why this should happen (a reasoned approached) (Tabachnick & Klien, 2011), with work having been done to consider how this is framed at a public, policy, and practice level (McCartan, Kemshall, & Tabachnick, 2015a, 2015b).

The acceptance of sexual abuse prevention, particularly the prevention of CSA, at a theoretical level differs from its acceptance at a policy and practice level. The theoretical and academic underpinnings are robust (Kemshall & McCartan, 2022; Smallbone et al, 2008), but the empirical research and practice evidence base is sporadic, small scale and difficult to replicate (Protect to prevent, 2025; Global Prevention, 2025; McCartan, 2024). The inconsistency in the research evidence base is really highlighted across a number of key domains.

- **Across the four prevention levels** (primary, secondary, tertiary, and quaternary) with tertiary (relapse prevention), followed primary (education and social level prevention) having the strongest evidence base. Whereas secondary (prevention with people at risk of committing a sexual offence) and quaternary (harm reaction and social inclusion) having the weakest evidence base. Conversely, quaternary has a slightly stronger practice base than secondary prevention. Additionally, a lot of the secondary prevention evidence is small scale with narrow and limited data sets, which makes it difficult for policy makers to implement. However, there is a growth in secondary prevention research (i.e., Global Prevention, 2know, prevent to protect, Together for Childhood, and Project Dunkle Feld) but these projects need more time to develop robust evidence underpinnings.
- **Across the four socio-ecological levels** (individual, interpersonal, community, and societal) with interventions at the individual level (individual treatment and prevention interventions) having the most robust evidenced base, and interpersonal (e.g., restorative justice), community (e.g., Circles of Support and Accountability), and societal (e.g., government policy) having more varied and, at times limited,

research and evidence base. Additionally, at the societal level the evidence base needs to be viewed from two different perspectives (a) Societal: National and (b) Societal: Global/transnational. It is important to recognise that research and evidence on sexual abuse prevention varies by country and global region, therefore viewing society as one homogenous mass is unhelpful to understanding sexual abuse, its prevention and our response to it.

- **Across indicators of context levels** (population, country, culture, and geography) the research and evidenced base demonstrates that the context of sexual abuse is an important contributor to the scale, scope and nature of that abuse, and therefore how we can work to prevent it. However not all social, cultural, population, and environmental contexts in respect to sexual abuse are understood equally or as transparently. Most of the research on sexual abuse is based on the global north (including Australia and New Zealand), Westernised (mainly Anglophone countries, although there is an increasing Francophone research and evidence base) countries. Additionally, within and across countries and places not all cultures, populations, and communities are equally researched and accessed, with most research (traditionally) focusing on mainstream communities.
- **Across offence type and "offender" population levels** with research and tending to focus on men in the criminal justice system who have committed contact sexual offences (although this is rapidly shifting over the last 30 years with an increased focus on online sexual abuse and harm). This means that the research evidence base is not equally focused on all aspects of sexual abuse with less research being done on certain populations (e.g., women who sexually offend), specific sexual offences (i.e., more research is done on CSA than adult rape), and certain peoples and culture (i.e., certain communities, cultures and social groups); this needs to be focussed upon if prevention all types of sexual offences addressed.

The sexual abuse research base is strongest for men convicted of sexual abuse offences in Northern hemisphere, anglophone countries, and when the research and practice community started to examine other prevention levels (especially secondary) they stated with the is population as well. Therefore, it is useful to consider whether research evidence that informs EpiCrim policy and practice is adequate and able to identify the knowledge that is needed at often a nuanced level to effectively inform policy and practice.

To develop robust evidence, base for sexual abuse within an EpiCrim framework consideration needs to be given to messages, interventions, and approaches at the prevention, socio-ecological, context and offence levels. In doing this (re)consideration needs to be given to what the main outcomes and Key Performance Indicators (KPI's) are. Historically, sexual abuse was framed within a criminal justice narrative which meant that outcomes were linked to re-offending, breach, recall, and other aspects of risk and risk management. With the shift to a health and wellbeing frame consideration needs to be given to harm reduction, social inclusion, behaviour change, and community integration, however these concepts are difficult to measure. To overcome these challenges there needs to be a conceptualisation of the successful outcomes linked to preventing and responding to sexual abuse, so that, appropriate and measurable outcomes linked to the four levels that criminal justice can be built. It is important to build appropriate research evaluations so that an EpiCrim approach to sexual abuse can be effectively measured and therefore commissioned by policy makers and practitioners. Across this book the evidence base will be cross examined across different prevention levels, socio-ecological levels, contexts and offence populations to try and establish how fit for purpose the evidence is, what they gaps are in the data and how an adequate multi-systemic response to this issue can be achieved.

Conclusions

The current chapter has explored the EpiCrim approach and its increasingly relevant and important framework for the conceptualisation of approaches to sexual abuse. Sexual abuse, in all its forms and with all its populations, is preventable, but to effectively engage different individuals, and communities, in prevention narratives and interventions changes in approach and social perspectives is needed. Sexual abuse is a criminological issue, but it is one that is routed in education, health, public health, and society. Sexual abuse is an individual, interpersonal, community, and societal issue, which needs a varied, multi-level response that can only be achieved through shared understanding, communication, engagement, and research.

References

Banyard, V. L., Edwards, K. M., Rizzo, A. J., Rothman, E. F., Greenberg, P., & Kearns, M. C. (2020). Improving social norms and actions to prevent sexual and intimate partner violence: A pilot study of the impact of green dot community on youth. *Journal of Prevention and Health Promotion, 1*(2), 183–211. https://doi.org/10.1177/2632077020966571

Bradley, A. (2017). *Trauma-informed practice: Exploring the role of adverse life experiences on the behaviour of offenders and the effectiveness of associated criminal justice strategies*. Doctoral thesis, Northumbria University. http://nrl.northumbria.ac.uk/36275/

Brennan, M., Perkins, D., Merdian, H., Tyrrell, E., Babchishin, K., mccartan, K. F., & Kelly, R. (2019). *Best practice in the management of online sex offending*. International Working

Brooke (2025). *Traffick light tool*. Accessible via https://www.brook.org.uk/education/sexual-behaviours-traffic-light-tool/

Brown, J. (2017). Public health, prevention and risk management. In K. Mccartan, & H. Kemshall (Eds) *Contemporary sex offender risk management, Volume I: Perceptions*. Palgrave Macmillian. Chapter 2.

Centres for Disease Control and Prevention (CDC). (2004). *Sexual violence prevention: Beginning the dialogue*. Retrieved 17 December 2020 fromhttp://www.cdc.gov/violenceprevention/pub/svprevention.html

Child light. (2024). Childlight: Global child safety insititue. Accessable via https://www.childlight.org/

Child light. (2025). Into the light index. Accessiable via https://intothelight.childlight.org/

Colding, J., & Barthel, S. (2019). Exploring the social-ecological systems discourse 20 years later. *Ecology and Society, 24*(1). https://www.jstor.org/stable/26796920

Di Gioia, R., & Beslay, L. (2023). *Help seeker and perpetrator prevention initiatives.*

Di Gioia, R., Besley, L., Cassar, A., & Pawula, A. (2022). *Classification criteria for child sexual abuse and exploitation prevention programmes.* JRC Technical Report. European Commission.

Di Gioia, R., Debnarovab, L., Beslayc, L., Lacambred, M., Miele, C., Quayle, E., Shaw, S., Xella, C., von Heyden, M., & mccartan, K. F. (in Press). Preventing and fighting child sexual abuse and exploitation: Current efforts and future directions in the European Union. *Victims and Offenders.*

Dworkin, E. R., Krahé, B., & Zinzow, H. (2021). The global prevalence of sexual assault: A systematic review of international research since 2010. *Psychology of Violence, 11*(5), 497–508.

ECPAT International (2024). *Scoping review of international approaches to child sexual abuse and exploitation prevention interventions by law enforcement.* ECPA International.

Ellefsen, H. B., Bjørkelo, B., Sunde, I. M., & Fyfe, N. R. (2023). Unpacking preventive policing: Towards a holistic framework. *International Journal of Police Science & Management, 25*(2), 196–207. https://doi.org/10.1177/14613557231163403

European Union (2021). *The costs of gender-based violence in the European Union.* European Union

Fisher-Kowalski, M. (2015). Social ecology. In J. D. Wright (Ed.), *International encyclopaedia of the social & behavioural sciences* (2nd ed., pp. 254–262). Elsevier.

Hackett, S. (2010) Children, young people and sexual violence. In C. Barter, & D. Berridge (eds) *Children behaving badly? Exploring peer violence between children and young people.* Blackwell Wiley.

Harris, D. A., Sheath, M., & Shields, R. (2024). First, do no harm: Critically revisiting contemporary approaches to child sexual abuse prevention. *Child Abuse & Neglect, 153.*https://doi.org/10.1016/j.chiabu.2024.106859

Hicks, J. (2021). *Global evidence on the prevalence and impact of online gender-based violence.* K4D Helpdesk Report. Institute of Development Studies. https://doi.org/10.19088/K4D.2021.140

HM Inspectorate of Probation (2025). Children displaying harmful sexual behaviour. Accessible via https://www.justiceinspectorates.gov.uk/hmiprobation/research/the-evidence-base-youth-offending-services/specific-sub-groups/children-displaying-harmful-sexual-behaviour/

Independent Inquiry into Child Sexual Abuse (2022). *The report of the independent inquiry into child sexual abuse: Attitudes to child sexual abuse.* Independent Inquiry into Child Sexual Abuse.

Karsna, K., & Bromley, P. (2024). *Child sexual abuse un 2022/23: Trends in the official data.* Centre for expertise in child sexual abuse.

Kemshall, H. (2017). The historical evolution of sex offender risk management. In K. mccartan, H. Kemshall (Eds.), *Contemporary sex offender management* (Vol. 1, pp. 205–230). Palgrave macmillan.

Kemshall, H., & Moulden, H. M. (2017). Communicating about Child Sexual Abuse with the Public: Learning the lessons from public awareness campaigns. *Journal of Sexual Aggression, 23*, 124–138. https://doi.org/10.1080/13552600.2016.1222004

Kemshall, H., & McCartan, K. F., (2022). *Desistance, recovery, and justice capital: Putting it all together.* HM Inspectorate of Probation.

King-Hill, S. (2022a). Child sexual abuse review: listening to children and young people is crucial. The conversation. Accessed via https://theconversation.com/child-sexual-abuse-review-listening-to-children-and-young-people-is-crucial-193356

King-Hill, S. (2022b). Knowledge translation and evidence-informed policy challenges: The implementation of the Brook Traffic Light Tool in Cornwall. *Journal of Sexual Aggression, 29*(2), 208–225. https://doi.org/10.1080/13552600.2022.2052770

King-Hill, S. (2023). The lost voice of boys in pastoral education. In Trotman, D., Jones, P., Purdy, N., & Tucker, S. (eds.*). Pastoral care in education: New directions for new times* (pp. 61–76 16). Cambridge Scholars Publishing.

King-Hill, S., McCartan, K. F., Gilsmann, A., Beavis, J., & Adams, A. (2023). *Understanding and Responding to Sibling Sexual Abuse*. Palgrave MacMillan.

King-Hill, S. (2024). *Executive summary: Young people's voices: Relationships, sex and health education.*

King-Hill, S., & mccartan, K. F. (2024). Good sex and relationships education can help teens understand when behaviour is abusive or controlling. *The Conversation Uk.*

Kitzinger, J. (2004). *Framing abuse: Media influence and public understanding of sexual violence against children.* Pluto Press.

Lainer, M. M. (2010). Epidemiological criminology (epicrim): Definition and application. *Journal of Theoretical and Philosophical Criminology, 2*(1), 63–103.

Letourneau, E. J., Eaton, W. W., Bass, J., Berlin, F. S., & Moore, S. G. (2014). The need for a comprehensive public health approach to preventing child sexual abuse. *Public Health Reports, 129*(3), 222–228.

Letourneau, E. (2024). *Building a new narrative on child sexual abuse prevention.* Psychology Today. Accessed via https://www.psychologytoday.com/gb/blog/prevention-now/202404/building-a-new-narrative-on-child-sexual-abuse-prevention

McCartan, K., & Gotch, K. (2020). International approaches to the management of perpetrators of sexual harm policy. In J. Proulx, F. Cortoni, L. Craig, & E. Letourneau (Eds.), *The Wiley handbook of what works with sexual offenders: Contemporary perspectives in theory, assessment, treatment, and prevention* (pp. 441–454). Wiley.

Mccartan, K., Uzieblo, K., & Smid, W. J. (2021). Professionals' understandings of and attitudes to the prevention of sexual abuse: An international exploratory study. *International Journal of Offender Therapy and Comparative Criminology, 65*, 815–831. https://doi.org/10.1177/0306624X20919706

McCartan, K. F. (2022). *Adapting out thinking on theory and practice in working with people convicted of a sexual offence.* HM Inspectorate of Probation.

McCartran, K. F. (2024). *Scoping review of international approaches to child sexual abuse and exploitation prevention interventions by law enforcement.* ECPAT International.

McCartan, K. F., & King-Hill, S. (2024). Developing a framework for the prevention of sibling sexual behaviour. *Child Abuse & Neglect*

McCartan, K. F., Kemshall, H., & Tabachnick, J. (2015a). The construction of community understandings of sexual violence: Rethinking public, practitioner and policy discourses. *Journal of Sexual Aggression, 21*(1), 100–116.

McCartan, K. F., Kemshall, H., & Tabachnick, J. (2015b). The reality of community understandings of sexual violence: Rethinking public, practitioner and policy discourses. *Journal of Sexual Aggression, 21*(1), 100–116.

McCartan, K., & Kemshall, H. (2023). Incorporating quaternary prevention: Understanding the full scope of public health practices in sexual abuse prevention. *International Journal of Offender Therapy and Comparative Criminology, 67*(2–3), 224–246. https://doi.org/10.1177/0306624X211049204

McGee, T., & Farrington, D. (2019). Developmental and life-course theories of crime. *Criminology & Criminal Justice Accessed at*. https://doi.org/10.1093/acrefore/9780190264079.013.250

Merdian, H. L., Perkins, D. E., Webster, S. D., & mccashin, D. (2019). Transnational child sexual abuse: Outcomes from a roundtable discussion. *International Journal of Environmental Research and Public Health, 16(2),* 243.

Meyrick, J. (2022). *#metoo for Women and Men: Understanding power through sexual harassment*. Taylor & Francis (Routledge).

Meyrick, J., McCartan, K. F., Eason, A., Curtis, B., & Rees, E. (2024). Across landscapes and lifespan: Causes and solutions of gender-based violence from survivors of sexual violence against women and girls (VAWG). *Journal of Sexual Aggression,* https://doi.org/10.1080/13552600.2024.2421197

NHS (2025). Definition of public health. Accessed via https://www.healthcareers.nhs.uk/working-health/working-public-health/what-public-health

NSPCC (2025). *Together for childhood*. Accessed via https://www.nspcc.org.uk/keeping-children-safe/our-services/together-for-childhood/

Prevention Global (2025). *Prevention global*. Accessed via https://www.prevention.global/

Pringer, S. M., & Wagner, N. J. (2020). Use of trauma-informed care with incarcerated offenders. *Journal of Addictions & Offender Counseling, 41*(1), 52–64. https://doi.org/10.1002/jaoc.12075

Protect children (2025). *Protect children.* https://www.suojellaanlapsia.fi/en/2know

Protech (2025). *Protech.* https://www.protechproject.eu/about

Protect and Prevent Through Support (2024). *Protect and prevent through support*. Retrieved February 29, 2024, from https://2ps-project.eu/

Proulx, J., Cortoni, F., Craig, L. A., & Letourneau, E. J. (2020). *The Wiley handbook of what works with sexual offenders: Contemporary perspectives in theory, assessment, treatment, and prevention.* Wiley.

Senker, S., Eason, A., Pawson, C., & mccartan, K. (2023). *Issues, challenges and opportunities for trauma-informed practice*. HMI Probation.

Smallbone, S., Marshall, W. L., & Wortley, R. (2008). *Preventing child sexual abuse: Evidence*. Willan Publishing.

Sutton, A., Cherney, A., White, R., & Clancey, G. (2021). *Crime prevention: Principles.* Cambridge University Press.

Tabachnick, J., & Klein, A. (2011). A *reasoned approach: Reshaping sex offender policy to prevent child sexual abuse*. Oregon: Association for the Treatment of Sexual Abusers.

Toates, F., Smid, W., & van der Berg, W. (2017). A framework for understanding sexual violence: Incentive-motivation and hierarchical control.

Aggression and Violent Behaviour, 34, 238–253. https://doi.org/10.1016/j.avb.2017.01.001

UNICEF. (2020). *Action to end child sexual abuse and exploitation: A review of the evidenc*e. UNICEF.

UNICEF. (2021). *Global annual results report 2021: Every child is protected from violence and exploitation.* UNICEF. Retrieved February 28, 2024, from https://www.unicef.org/reports/global-annual-results-2021-goal-area-3

UNICEF. (nd.). *Brief on the social ecological model.* UNICEF. Retrieved February 25, 2024, from chrome-extension://efaidnbmnnnibpcajpcglclefindmkaj/; https://www.unicef.org/media/135011/file/Global%20multisectoral%20operational%20framework.pdf

United Nations. (2014). *United Nations model strategies and practical measures on the elimination of violence against children in the field of crime prevention and criminal justice.* United Nations, General Assembly, A/C.3/69/L.5*.

United Nations. (2020). *No country is free from child sexual abuse, exploitation, UN's Top Rights Forum Hears.* UN News, 3 March 2020. Retrieved February 25, 2024, from https://news.un.org/en/story/2020/03/1058501

United Nations (2022). *United Nations rights of the child*. United Nations. Accessed via https://www.unicef.org.uk/what-we-do/un-convention-child-rights/

United Nations. (2024). *The UN guidelines for the prevention of crime.* United Nations. Retrieved February 25, 2024, from https://www.unodc.org/unodc/en/justice-and-prison-reform/cpcj-crimeprevention-home.html

United Nations (2025). *Sexual violence.* United Nations. Accessed via https://dataunodc.un.org/data/crime/sexual-violence

Uzieblo, K., Smid, W. J., & McCartan, K. F. (2022). *Challenges in the management of people convicted of a sexual offence. A way forward*. Palgrave Macmillan.

Victim Commissioner (2021). ONS survey reveals just one in six female rape victims report to the police. Victim Commissioner. Accessed via https://victimscommissioner.org.uk/news/ons-survey-march-2020/

Wager, N., Myers, A., & Parkinson, D. (2021). *Police disruption of child sexual abuse: A scoping review.* Centre foe expertise on child sexual abuse.

Wilson, R., Sandler, J., & McCartan, K. F. (2020). Community dynamic risk management of persons who have sexually offended. In J. Proulx, F. Cortoni, L. A. Craig, & E. J. Letourneau (Eds.), *The wiley handbook of what works with sexual offenders: Contemporary perspectives in theory, assessment, treatment, and prevention.* Wiley. Chapter 14.

3

What Can "EpiCrim" Approaches Contribute to the Effective Multi-Agency Management of High Risk Offenders in the Community?

Hazel Kemshall

Introduction

Recent years have seen an increased focus on "EpiCrim" approaches to managing offenders in the community. This has included high risk offenders, particularly, but not exclusively, sex offenders. This chapter will review the critical ingredients of such an approach and how it might assist existing multi-agency public protection arrangements for the community management of sexual and violent offenders. The chapter will recommend both policy and practical changes that are likely to enhance the effective use of "EpiCrim" in multi-agency responses, including how the UK Multi-Agency Public Protection Arrangements (MAPPA) might benefit from such an approach and how the use of an EpiCrim informed approach might strengthen and complement multi-agency work. In particular, the shift from largely reactive responses to

H. Kemshall (✉)
De Montfort University, Leicester, UK
e-mail: hazelkemshall@gmail.com

K. McCartan et al. (eds.), *Developing and Implementing a Public Health and Criminological Approach to Tackling Sexual Abuse*, Palgrave Studies in Risk, Crime and Society, https://doi.org/10.1007/978-3-031-93634-0_3

offending towards an "upstream" approach of increased prevention work within communities could have both societal and financial benefits going forward, particularly important as we enter another age of austerity. The chapter will include "helpful hints" for those policy makers, managers and practitioners keen to adopt an "EpiCrim" approach in multi-agency settings.

What Is "EpiCrim"?

EpiCrim is the application of public health preventive approaches to criminology and finding practical ways to apply epidemiological preventive approaches to real crime problems, for example sexual offending (Rowhani-Rahbar & Hannah, 2024). In addition, EpiCrim utilises both a multi-disciplinary and multi-agency approach to crime prevention and reduction, working across disciplinary boundaries and promoting interagency work to formulate and implement practical strategies (see Lanier, 2010). An EpiCrim approach focuses strongly on prevention rather than mere reaction after the fact of offending (for a discussion of the four levels of prevention please see Chapter 1).

This prevention model has also been applied to violent offending (McCartan & Kemshall, 2023).

The model also recognises and relies upon the socio-ecological model of crime (McCartan & Kemshall, 2021; McCartan & Richards, 2021). The socio-ecological model theorises that sex offending, but also other harmful offending, is best understood by considering the subtle combination of individual factors such as predispositions and personality traits; relationship factors such as intimate family relationships, being in abusive relationships or environments; community factors such as spaces, places and contexts that afford access to victims and harmful offending; and societal factors such as cultural norms of acceptability, gender inequality, lack of concern and visibility for particular crimes (McCartan, 2022).

Whilst single interventions may address only one of the above areas, EpiCrim advocates that such interventions are more effective if combined and "joined up" into coherent, integrated approaches to crime prevention and reduction. For example, joining up person centred interventions to change thinking patterns and propensities to offend with positive interventions into the family and relationship arena to reduce abusive environments; and combining these with environmental and community management strategies to reduce access to places, spaces and victims (e.g. criminals record checking, barring from key professions, and mandatory reporting of abuse); and public awareness campaigns to promote societal awareness and evidence based policy responses to harmful offending (Kemshall & Moulden, 2017).

EpiCrim and Multi-Agency Public Protection Arrangements (MAPPA)

One arena where the use of EpiCrim could be further considered is in the Multi-Agency Public Protection Arrangements (MAPPA). These arrangements are used across the UK to manage high risk sexual and violent offenders in the community, with more recent extension across European countries (see Kemshall & Hilder, 2020). In brief, MAPPA comprises police, prisons and probation/criminal justice social work agencies as the main partners, with other agencies such as social services and housing as "Duty to Cooperate" partners.

The aim of MAPPA is to provide multi-agency panels to carry out multi-agency risk assessment and risk management planning, and to gain access to a wide range of resources required to effectively manage risky and challenging people in the community, including on discharge from prison (see Kemshall, 2019; Kemshall & Hilder, 2020, for a full review). At present, MAPPA largely focuses on person centred interventions to mitigate risky behaviours, treatments to change thinking patterns and decision making, and controlling measures to reduce access to victims (Kemshall, 2018; Wood & Kemshall, 2007).

Research over the last 20 years have shown MAPPA to be effective with helpful reductions in sexual offending in particular amongst those subject to the MAPPA (Bryant et al., 2015; Criminal Justice Inspectorates, 2022; Peck, 2011). However, the Criminal Justice Inspectorates report (2022) noted that local area MAPPAs could be challenged by restricted resources, that there were "gaps" and inconsistencies in practice, and the transition from custody to community did not always receive the necessary MAPPA oversight. Whilst the report noted considerable positive improvements overtime and a real contribution to the reduction of harmful violent and sexual offending, what is clear is that MAPPA on its own cannot be the sole answer to crime reduction and prevention of harmful offending. It is therefore helpful to consider the following:

- What other strategies for crime prevention and crime reduction may be helpful.
- How MAPPA might contribute to, and influence, alternative strategies.

The following sections will consider these issues.

Alternative Strategies and the Role of MAPPA

The levels of prevention outlined above have been researched and evaluated over recent years (CDC, 2015). This has resulted in a more refined view of how the prevention levels actually operate in practice; and most notably that the levels of prevention tend to overlap and boundaries between them are permeable (Letourneau, 2017). Prevention responses have become more sophisticated over time. For example, the *Enough Abuse* public awareness campaign in Massachusetts operates across all three prevention levels by:

- developing and delivering broad based educational/training courses aimed at preventing victimisation and encouraging early recognition and disclosure of sexual offending behaviour or grooming for primary prevention
- enabling and training on self-risk management techniques for perpetrators at the secondary level, advocating for mandatory reporting, and organisational checking and disclosure

- phone lines to enable perpetrator and victim disclosure and "help seeking" at tertiary level, including on-going support to victims, and promulgation of effective treatments and interventions to prevent reoffending.

(Massachusetts Citizens for Children, 2010; Schrober et al., 2012a, 2012b).

Subject to resource constraints MAPPA locally and at national level could input critical advice and expertise to such initiatives, particularly on educational content; the best self-risk management techniques to focus on; how best to manage spaces and places where offending can occur; and the promulgation of effective interventions and treatments. Working alongside organisations involved in these types of initiatives could also help to close the gap between "communities of interest" and professionals working with harmful perpetrators and provide professionals with a window onto wider public concerns. This can help to reduce negative public perceptions and hostility to the professional management of high risk persons in the community (Kemshall & Moulden, 2017). Arguably this would enable greater access to "lay person" views than can be provided by the use of individual lay advisors currently.

The UPSTREAM project in Scotland led by Stop It Now! is another example of sexual offence prevention, with the name reflecting the focus on stopping sexual offending before it happens (see: www.theupstreamproject.org.uk; accessed May 23rd 2024). The project comprises online resources for use by professionals and members of the public to learn, teach and train about sexual offence prevention. This is an example of primary level prevention and follows effective messaging principles (Health Development Agency, 2004) by focusing on "know, learn, identify, prevent, and act". It can assist professionals to improve prevention of reoffending and early detection at the secondary level; and increases community knowledge and involvement in prevention. As such, it can work alongside MAPPA and assist in local crime reduction.

The Criminal Justice Inspectorate report on MAPPA (2022) found particular difficulties for MAPPA level 1 cases. In brief, those cases managed by a single agency, and often without additional resources. Case workers felt challenged, and at times distanced from the MAPPA process, working with risky people without, on occasion, sufficient skill, expertise or knowledge. Access to tried and tested resources for community interventions could provide part of the answer, providing additional knowledge and confidence to police and probation officers carrying these caseloads.

At the community and societal levels, EpiCrim can provide useful population level data to assist in formulating crime prevention policies and initiatives. For example, to identify who in the population are the main perpetrators and with what profiles and risk factors. This can aid early identification for help and support; who in the population are most "at risk", where and why, in order to assist in planning outreach work and effective messaging on safety, and resource distribution across locales and contexts (Rice et al., 2013). Whilst Chicago, Los Angeles and Philadelphia have used such data to target neighbourhoods for policing violent crime, more recent evaluative research has indicated that over policing and arrest rates in themselves can have a detrimental impact over time, leading to resentment and diminishing returns, principally because social conditions do not change, and underlying causation factors remain (Muchow, 2023).

Overtime the public health approach is lost, and the focus on understanding and addressing the underlying causal factors fades. Interventions become reactive rather than responsive. Within the UK key cities have pursued a similar use of epidemiological data and crime prevention techniques, principally Merseyside (www.merseysidevrp.com); London (www.london.gov.uk/content/londons-violence-reduction-unit); and the Violence Reduction Programme in Scotland (http://www.svru.co.uk/).

The Scottish Violence Reduction Unit uses a public health approach to understand and address the underlying causes of violence. In addition to a range of projects the SVRU is committed to research and evaluations, offering key summaries for practitioners, and rapid reviews of the available research evidence for example on youth violence, and also on knife crime. Importantly, the overall approach recognises that simply striving to "fix individuals" without understanding and addressing social and environmental factors is likely to have limited impact (Linden, 2023). As Linden states: "We need to think much more holistically to consider the real-world environment, how the problem of violence is created and how it is sustained". (Linden, 2023: 145).

Epidemiological data might help national and local MAPPA to consider more holistic approaches, as well as identify locales from which violent and/or sexual crime is likely to emanate or result in repeat victimisation. This information could both influence local MAPPA strategies, for example on communicating with "at risk communities", but also influence resource allocation.

EpiCrim and the public health approach it utilises also encourages a policy and practice focus on long-term change, thus diminishing repeat offending and repeat victimisation. This aim has resulted in increased practice and research attention to what has been labelled as "quaternary prevention", that is an additional fourth level to the earlier three tier approach to prevention. In the crime arena, this has aided a useful link to desistance supportive work, and those life course and social condition changes that are likely to result in long-term change for the better (McCartan & Kemshall, 2023; Tesser, 2017). Arguably, quaternary prevention sets an ambitious agenda for future work with those who commit harmful offending, particularly on how to achieve and sustain a risk-free life and achieve positive and supportive reintegration into communities that can be hostile and unwelcoming. The next section explores some of the key issues.

Quaternary Prevention: Being Ambitious for the Future

Quaternary prevention encourages a focus on interventions designed to achieve long-term offence free lives, pro-social identities, and positive integration into the community (McCartan & Kemshall, 2023). Specific intervention "ingredients" are seen as critical to quaternary prevention, in particular desistance focused practice; long-term reintegration post custody utilising a range of skills and competences (often referred to as "recovery capital"); and trauma informed practice (see: Best, 2019; CDC, 2004; McCartan & Gotch, 2020; McCartan & Kemshall, 2020). Arguably a greater focus on quaternary prevention would ensure that post custody reintegration would receive increased policy and practice attention, helping to break the cycle of victimisation and reducing perpetrator activities. At present the sustainability of risk-free lives is challenging (Best & Colman, 2019; Best et al., 2018), and the practice and policy gaze is restricted to immediate release and resettlement. MAPPA, particularly at the level of the Responsible Authority National Steering Group (RANSG), could potentially make an important contribution here by:

- providing data on local and national housing/accommodation trends in order to make an evidenced case for additional resources and support
- collecting data on where stigma and community hostility has undermined reintegration, collecting and disseminating best practice MAPPA responses to these challenges
- contributing to a policy agenda aimed at achieving effective longer-term reintegration of those who have committed harmful offending.

At MAPPA national level the RANSG, and at local level MAPPA Strategic Management Groups or Strategic Oversight Groups, could take a leadership role in ensuring a just and proportionate approach to offender management is adopted, including explicitly seeking and quality assuring approaches that balance risks, rights and reintegration (Kemshall, 2017, 2019; McCartan, Kemshall & Hoggett, 2017). Local quality assurance coupled with a national (possibly an inspection) focus on proportionality in the use of interventions and controls/conditions would arguably strengthen attention to ethics, rights and proportionality in practice (Fenton, 2013; Mann et al., 2018; Maruna & Mann, 2019). Overly precautionary practice would be discouraged (Lippke, 2008), curtailing an incremental drift into the "preventive state" (Janus, 2006; Slobogin, 2011).

Other jurisdictions are beginning to explore alternative management strategies and framing approaches to achieve crime prevention without creating a "preventive state". For example, New Zealand has reframed their sex offender register into a mechanism for the delivery of strengths-based interventions and supportive reintegration into communities (McCartan & Laws, 2018; McCartan & Kemshall, 2023). Whilst the New Zealand approach is still under on-going evaluation, it is an interesting example of quaternary prevention in action, and an example of "supportive authority" and long-term scrutiny with positive integration at its heart. Barnes and Law have described it as: "strengths-based case management practice which balances the need to manage risk, with the needs of the person on the register" (2019: 27). This is in sharp contrast to the UK system where the sex offender register and case management are in reality separated, and the register inadvertently functions as a stigmatising and socially isolating process (McCartan & Kemshall, 2023; O'Sullivan et al., 2016).

The Responsible Authority National Steering Group (RANSG) and local MAPPA Steering Groups/Strategic Oversight Groups could play a key role in encouraging the greater use of desistance supportive work in MAPPA risk management planning, enabling practitioners to integrate rehabilitative strategies alongside community protection measures (Kemshall, 2019). Such strategies seek a balanced approach to risk management focusing on desistance and rehabilitation; changing risky behaviours and meeting legitimate needs; reducing risks and reducing reoffending behaviours; and avoiding over-intrusion on those whose risk does not justify it (Kemshall, 2021: 4). This approach has been called "blended protection" (Kemshall, 2008) and offers a balanced and proportionate response to risk and rehabilitation. However, "being soft on sex offenders" (and violent offenders) opens practitioners and policy makers to significant levels of public criticism, rejection, and moral repugnance (Harper & Hogue, 2015; Harper et al., 2017; Stafford & Vandiver, 2017). Therefore, seeking to change public and media perceptions is important.

Local MAPPA can play a key role in doing this. For example, through annual reports and showcasing individual success stories that promulgate safe reintegration and desistance as routes to risk reduction. In addition, other more innovatory methods are already being explored, for example short videos for social media; educational films for public consumption;

messages directed at community "opinion formers" such as elected representatives and leaders of community groups. Dissemination to schools, parent groups, voluntary community groups and faith groups have all been seen as key routes to influencing public perceptions with reasonable levels of effectiveness (Kemshall & Moulden, 2017).

Working through "opinion formers" and existing groups of influence has greater impact than "mass media" campaigns, where much of the message is lost or resisted (see Kemshall & Moulden, 2017 for a full discussion). Extensive research indicates that the following is helpful for effective communication with communities and public:

- Importance of social networks and context in opinion formation (Kemshall & Moulden, 2017), particularly existing groups of influence who help to frame local public opinion. These can be family networks, employment networks, leisure, and faith groups. They can be useful in gaining access to communities, and in framing messages effectively.
- Messages are mediated and understood through existing beliefs and existing schemas, and whether the recipient has the self-belief and self-efficacy to act on what they are told (Kitzinger, 1999). Listening is active not passive, and hearers of the message tend to test the content against existing beliefs. Thus, understanding belief systems can be fundamental to framing messages and increasing their impact and receptivity.
- Vivid risks are the most feared (Slovic, 2016); this includes public perceptions of sex crimes (Critcher, 2011; Stafford & Vandiver, 2017).
- Risk inflation is usually due to lack of trust, and often is an addition to existing fears and anxieties (Slovic, 2016). Risk management failures and "Serious Incidents" with their subsequent media coverage erode public trust, and cumulatively over time can reduce public confidence to a low ebb, even in those areas where failures have not occurred. Erosion of trust in professionals and the formal risk management system becomes "contagious". This contributes to a distancing effect and fuels vigilantism (Kemshall, 2008).

- Maximise the relevance of the message to the audience using tried and tested techniques and accessible language (Health Development Agency, 2004; TDI, 2007).
- Maximise audience perception of susceptibility to the risk; i.e. that the risk matters to them even if they themselves may not be directly harmed by it (Bohner & Wanke, 2009; CDC, 2004; Massachusetts Citizens for Children, 2010).
- Give a clear message about the benefits of acting on the message, i.e. greater personal and community safety (Bohner & Wanke, 2009).
- The message should promote self-efficacy and key actions that can be taken by the individual, for example a "what do message if you see X" (Kemshall, 2008; Tabachnick & Newton-Ward, 2010; TDI, 2007; see also Health Development Agency, 2004).
- Avoid "generalised anxiety" and use "functional fear" (Jackson & Gray, 2010; Kemshall & Weaver, 2012). Generalised anxiety stems from messages that leave the hearer without help, support or clear messages about actions to take, thus creating a sense of anxiety. Functional fear stems from messages that enable listeners to do something about the risk. Crime prevention messages about locks, windows, dwelling house safety measures are a clear example of effective functional fear messages.

Local MAPPA Strategic Management Boards or Strategic Oversight Groups could ensure that all or some of these strategies are adopted in order to improve communication with communities and public, thus creating better conditions for community management and long-term reintegration of persons under their oversight.

Conclusion

EpiCrim has the potential to offer much to crime prevention and reduction. Exciting and innovatory projects have been initiated in recent years utilising this approach and the continuum of prevention levels as described in early research (e.g. Lanier, 2010). Some of these projects have also focused on evaluative research of their activities, adding to our understanding and refining the EpiCrim model over time.

The recent addition of quaternary prevention has added important concerns about ethics, and rights, and the sustainability of interventions and change for the long-term, and the creation of more accepting and tolerant communities for the reintegration journey. In addition, quaternary prevention enables a focus on community-based initiatives alongside person centred interventions, providing for more holistic responses to the problem of sexual and violent offending. There is also much to gain from epidemiological data, particularly on population level risks and vulnerabilities, and on those places and spaces most likely to lead to repeat offending and repeat victimisation.

For MAPPA EpiCrim has relevance at both the strategic and operational levels. At the strategic level EpiCrim could help inform:

- Resource allocation and targeting using epidemiological data; especially to aid the management of places and spaces as well as individuals.
- Improved communication strategies and techniques, using methods tried and tested in the public health sphere, and in public health campaigns against sexual offending and violent crime.
- Setting quality assurance standards for ethical practice and the preservation of rights.
- Seeking greater input to, and alignment with, public health campaigns and initiatives on sexual and violent crime prevention.

At the MAPPA operational level existing EpiCrim projects, data and research could assist with the following:

- Providing access to prevention "tool kits" and training resources that case workers would benefit from, thus filling the skill and competence gap quickly and relatively cheaply for the lone practitioner in the key risk management agencies of police and probation/criminal justice social work.
- Promotion of effective desistance supportive work alongside risk management planning, with a particular focus on custody to community transitions.

- Greater attention to the long-term, particularly resilient and sustainable reintegration; including plans to gain and sustain recovery capital, deliver trauma reducing interventions, and gain greater community embeddedness for those who are disconnected from communities.
- Consideration of rights and ethical practice when formulating risk management plans, and actively discouraging overly precautionary practice.

EpiCrim is an idea whose time has come, not least because the cost of crime management is challenging, and reactive measures alone cannot produce enough effectiveness for the economic costs incurred (Saied-Tessier, 2014). Undoubtedly, MAPPA has improved its performance levels since its inception in 1998 and increased its overall effectiveness in preventing repeat offending and repeat victimisation. However, it is only one part of what could be a much broader and effective crime prevention picture. A crime prevention picture framed by EpiCrim principles, methods and values; combining "upstream" interventions at one end of the prevention continuum with quaternary prevention methods to ensure "Good Lives" at the other. MAPPA can both gain from, and contribute to, the EpiCrim agenda on crime prevention.

References

Best, D. (2019) *Pathways to recovery and desistance: The role of the social contagion of hope.* Policy Press.

Best, D., & Colman, C. (2019). *Strengths-Based approaches to crime and substance use.* Routledge.

Best, D., Musgrove, A., & Hall, L. (2018). The bridge between social identity and community capital on the path to recovery and desistance. *Probation Journal, 65*(4), 394–406.

Bohner, G., & Wanke, M. (2009). The psychology of attitudes and persuasion. In J. Wood & T. Gannon (Eds.), *Public opinion and criminal justice* (pp. 3–32). Willan.

Bryant, S., Peck, M., & Lovbakke, J. (2015) *Reoffending analysis of MAPPA eligible offenders.* Ministry of Justice (UK). Retrieved May 22, 2024, from https://www.gov.uk/government/uploads/system/uploads/attachment_data/file/407139/reoffending-analysis-of-mappa-eligible-offenders.pdf

Centers for Disease Control and Prevention (CDC) (2004) *Sexual violence prevention: Beginning the dialogue*. Retrieved December 17, 2020; May 22, 2024 from http://www.cdc.gov/violenceprevention/pub/svprevention.html

Centers for Disease Control and Prevention (CDC). (2015). *The social-ecological model: A framework for prevention.* Last updated March, 2015; Retrieved 22, 2024, from http://www.cdc.gov/violenceprevention/overview/social-ecologicalmodel.html

Criminal Justice Inspectorates (2022) *Twenty years on, is MAPPA achieving its objectives? A joint thematic inspection of multi-agency public protection arrangements.* Retrieved May 22, 2024, from www.justiceinspectorates.gov.uk/hmiprobation/inspections/mappa-thematic/

Critcher, C. (2011). A political economy of moral panics. *Crime, Media, Culture: An International Journal, 7*(3), 2024. https://doi.org/10.1177/1741659011417605(AccessedMay23rd

Fenton, J. (2013). Risk aversion and anxiety in Scottish criminal justice social work: Can desistance and human rights agendas have an impact? *The Howard Journal of Criminal Justice, 52*(1), 77–90.

Harper, C. A., & Hogue, T. E. (2015). The emotional representation of sexual crime in the national British press. *Journal of Language and Social Psychology, 34*, 3–24.

Harper, C. A., Hogue, T. E., & Bartels, R. M. (2017). Attitudes towards sexual offenders: What do we know, and why are they important? *Aggression and Violent Behavior, 34*, 201–213.

Health Development Agency. (2004). The effectiveness of public health campaigns (HDA Briefing No. 7).

Jackson, J., & Gray, E. (2010). Functional fear and public insecurities about crime. *British Journal of Criminology, 50*, 1–22. https://doi.org/10.1093/bjc/azp059

Janus, E. (2006). *Failure to protect: America's sexual predator laws and the rise of the preventive state*. Cornell University Press.

Kemshall, H. (2008). *Understanding the community management of high risk offenders.* Open University McGraw Hill.

Kemshall, H. (2017). The historical evolution of sex offender risk management. In K. McCartan & H. Kemshall (Eds.), *Contemporary sex offender management* (Vol. 1, pp. 205–230). Palgrave MacMillan.

Kemshall, H. (2018). The rise of risk in probation work: Historical reflections and future speculations. In P. Priestley & Vanstone, M (Eds.), *Probation and Politics: Academic Reflections from Former Practitioners*. Palgrave.

Kemshall, H. (2019). A critical review of risk assessment policy and practice since the 1990s, and the contribution of risk practice to contemporary rehabilitation of offenders. In P. Ugwudike, H. Graham, F. McNeill, P. Raynor, F. S. Taxman & C. Trotter (Eds.), *The routledge companion to rehabilitative work in criminal justice*. Chapter 19. Routledge.

Kemshall, H. (2021). *Risk and desistance: A blended approach to risk management*. HMIProbation, Academic Insights 2021/07. Retrieved May 22, 2024, from www.justiceinspectorates.gov.uk/hmiprobation/wp-content/uploads/sites/5/2021/06/Academic-Insights-Kem

Kitzinger, J. (1999). Researching risk and the media. *Health, Risk & Society, 1*(1), 55–69.

Kemshall, H., & Hilder, S. (2020) Effective systems and processes for managing violent offenders in the United Kingdom and the European Union. In S. Wormith, A. C. Leam & E. H. Todd (Eds.), *The Wiley handbook of what works in violence risk management: Theory, research and practice*. Wiley. Retrieved May 21, 2024, from. https://doi.org/10.1002/9781119315933.ch25

Kemshall, H., Mackenzie, G., Wood, J., Bailey, R., & Yates, J. (2005) *Strengthening Multi-Agency Public Protection Arrangements (MAPPAs)*. Home Office Development and Practice Report, 45. Home Office.

Kemshall, H., & Moulden, H. M. (2017). Communicating about child sexual abuse with the public: learning the lessons from public awareness campaigns. *Journal of Sexual Aggression, 23*(2), 124–138. Retrieved May 21, 2024, from https://doi.org/10.1080/13552600.2016.1222004

Kemshall, H., & Weaver, B. (2012). The sex offender public disclosure pilots in England and Scotland: Lessons for 'marketing strategies' and risk communication with the public. *Criminology and Criminal Justice, 12*(5), 549–565.

Kitzinger, J. (1999). Researching risk and the media. *Health, Risk and Society, 1*(1), 55–69. Retrieved May 23, 2024, from https://doi.org/10.1080/13698579908407007

Lanier, M. (2010). Epidemiological criminology (EpiCrim): Definition and application. *Journal of Theoretical and Philosophical Criminology, 2*(1), 63–103. Retrieved May 21, 2024, from http://hdl.handle.net/10484/5226

Letourneau, E. (2017). *Watch my TEDMED talk on child sexual abuse prevention: Prevention is the only way to end victimization.*

Psychology Today. Retrieved January 27 2021; Retrieved May 22, 2024, from https://www.psychologytoday.com/intl/blog/prevention-now/201709/watch-my-tedmed-talkchild-sexual-abuse-prevention

Linden, W. (2023). Why a smörgåsbord of interventions won't solve violence: an applied public health approach to violence reduction in Scotland. *The International Journal of Forensic Psychotherapy, 5*(2), 145–148. Retrieved May 23, 2024, https://doi.org/10.33212/ijfp.v5n2.2023.145

Lippke, R. (2008). Response to tudor: Remorse-based sentence reductions in theory and practice. *Criminal Law and Philosophy, 2*, 259–268.

Mann, R., Howard, F., & Tew, J. (2018). What is a rehabilitative prison culture? *Prison Service Journal, 235*, 3–10.

Martins, C., Godycki-Cwirko, M., Heleno, B., & Brodersen, J. (2018). Quaternary prevention: Reviewing the concept. *European Journal of General Practice, 24*(1), 106–111.

Maruna, S., & Mann, R. (2019). *Reconciling 'Desistance' and 'what works'. HMIP academic insights 2019/1*. Manchester; HMIP. Retrieved May 22, 2024, from https://www.justiceinspectorates.gov.uk/hmiprobation/wp-content/uploads/sites/5/2019/02/Academic-Insights-Maruna-and-Mann-Feb-19-final.pdf

Massachusetts Citizens for Children. (2010). *Enough abuse campaign: Join the movement.* Retrieved May 23, 2024, www.enoughabuse.org/index.php?option=com_contentandview=articleandid=18andItemid=22

McCartan, K. (2022) Refining processes in policy and practice in working with people accused or convicted of a sexual offence. HMIProbation, Academic Insights 2022/01. Retrieved May 23, 2024, from www.justiceinspectorates.gov.uk/hmiprobation/wp-content/uploads/sites/5/2022/01/Academic-Insights-McCartan.pdf

McCartan, K., & Gotch, K. (2020). International approaches to the management of perpetrators of sexual Harm policy. In J. Proulx, F. Cortoni, L. Craig, & E. Letourneau (Eds.), *The Wiley Handbook of what works with sexual offenders: Contemporary perspectives in theory, assessment, treatment, and prevention* (pp. 441–454). Wiley.

McCartan, K., & Kemshall, H. (2020). The potential role of recovery capital in stopping sexual offending: Lessons from circles of support and accountability to enrich practice. *Irish Probation Journal, 17*, 87–106.

McCartan, K., & Kemshall, H. (2023) Incorporating quaternary prevention: Understanding the full scope of public health practices in sexual abuse prevention. *International Journal of Offender Therapy and Comparative Criminology; 2023 Feb; 67*(2–3), 224–246. Published online 2021 Oct

10. Retrieved May 22, 2024, from https://doi.org/10.1177/0306624X2110 49204

McCartan K., Kemshall H., & Hoggett J. (2017). Reframing the sex offender register and disclosures: From monitoring and control to desistance. In H. Kemshall, & K. McCartan (Eds.), *Contemporary sex offender risk management* (Vol. 2, pp. 205–231). Palgrave MacMillan.

McCartan, K., & Laws, M. A. (2018). Risk assessment and management of perpetrators of sexual abuse in New Zealand. *Sex Offender Treatment, 13*(1/ 2). Retrieved May 21, 2024, from http://www.sexual-offender-treatment. org/174.html

McCartan K, and Richards K. (2021) The Integration of People Convicted of a Sexual Offence Into the Community and Their (Risk) Management. *Curr Psychiatry Rep. 2021 Jul 1;23*(8), 52. Retrieved May 23, 2024, from https://doi.org/10.1007/s11920-021-01258-4. PMID: 34196851; PMCID: PMC8249282

Muchow, A. N. (2023). Community-oriented policing and violent crime: Evidence from the Los Angeles community safety partnership. *Police Quarterly, 26*(4), 545–572. Retrieved May 23, 2024, from https://doi.org/10. 1177/10986111231162353

O'Sullivan, J., Hoggett, H., McCartan, K. F., & Kemshall, H. (2016). Understandings, implications and alternative approaches to the use of the sex offenders register in the UK. *Irish Probation Journal, 13*, 84–101.

Peck, M. (2011) Patterns of reconviction among offenders eligible for Multi-Agency Public Protection Arrangements (MAPPA). Ministry of Justice Research Series 6/11. Retrieved May 22, 2024, from https://www.gov. uk/government/uploads/system/uploads/attachment_data/file/217373/pat terns-reconviction-mappa.pdf

Rice, C., Lee, S., Meza, M., & Fraser, C. (2013). A call to action: Los Angeles' quest to achieve community safety. Advancement project. Retrieved May 23, 2024, from http://www.advancementproject.org/resources/entry/a-call-to-action-los-angeles-quest-toachieve-community-safety

Rowhani-Rahbar, A., & Hannah, H. (2024) *Epidemiological criminology*. Oxford Research Encyclopaedias. https://doi.org/10.1093/acrefore/978019 0264079.013.847

Saied-Tessier, A. (2014). Estimating the costs of child sexual abuse in the UK. NSPCC, 1–44. Retrieved January 27, 2021, from https://www.nspcc.org. uk/globalassets/documents/research-reports/estimating-costs-child-sexual-abuse-uk.pdf (Accessed May 23rd, 2024).

Schober, D. J., Fawcett, S. B., & Bernier, J. (2012a). The enough abuse campaign: Building the movement to prevent child sexual abuse in Massachusetts. *Journal of Child Sexual Abuse, 21*, 456–469.

Schober, D. J., Fawcett, S. B., Thigpen, S., Curtis, A., & Wright, R. (2012b). An empirical case study of a child sexual abuse prevention initiative in Georgia. *Health Education Journal, 71*, 291–298.

Slobogin, C. (2011). Prevention of sexual violence by those who have been sexually violent. *International Journal of Law and Psychiatry, 34*, 210–216.

Slovic, P. (2016). The perception of risk. In: S. J. Sternberg, S. T. Fiske, & D. J. Foss (Eds.), *Scientists making a difference* (pp. 179–182). https://doi.org/10.1017/CBO9781316422250.040

Stafford M. C., & Vandiver D. M. (2017). Public perceptions of sex crimes and sex offenders. In T. Sanders (Ed.), *The Oxford Handbook of sex offences and sex offenders. Oxford Handbook online*. https://www.oxfordhandbooks.com/view/https://doi.org/10.1093/oxfordhb/9780190213633.001.0001/oxfordhb-9780190213633-e-25

Tabachnick, J., & Newton-Ward, M. (2010). *Using social marketing for effective sexual violence prevention. The prevention of sexual violence: A practitioner's sourcebook*. NEARI Press.

TDI (The Derwent Initiative). (2007). *Tackling sex offending together*. Newcastle upon Tyne: TDI. Retrieved May 22, 2024, www.tdi.org.uk

Tesser, C. D. (2017). Why is quaternary prevention important in prevention? *Revista de Saude Publica, 51*, 116. https://doi.org/10.11606/S1518-8787.2017051000041

Wood, J. & Kemshall, H. (2007) *The operation and experience of Multi-Agency Public Protection Arrangements (MAPPA)*. Home Office. Retrieved May 22, 2024, from http://www.dmu.ac.uk/documents/health-and-life-sciences-documents/research/rdsolr1207.pdf

4

Data Governance for Research Using Sensitive Data

Elizabeth Green and Felix Ritchie

Introduction

Research often requires the use of Personally Identifiable Information (PII), which has strict ethical and legal guidelines on how it can be collected, analysed and used. For Epidemiological Criminology (EpiCrim), this is particularly problematic because its subject matter, health and criminal activity, are two of the most sensitive pieces of personal information to work with. Indeed, health is a 'protected characteristic' under the General Data Protection Regulation (GDPR),[1] meaning additional measures should be taken to ensure use is fair,

[1] Although the GDPR formally only applies to countries in the Single European Market, it is widely seen as a model for good practice and is the basis for many regulations, such as the UK Data Protection Act 2018. We will use it in this chapter as a shorthand for 'modern principles-based regulation'.

E. Green · F. Ritchie (✉)
University of the West of England, Bristol, UK
e-mail: felix.ritchie@uwe.ac.uk

K. McCartan et al. (eds.), *Developing and Implementing a Public Health and Criminological Approach to Tackling Sexual Abuse*, Palgrave Studies in Risk, Crime and Society, https://doi.org/10.1007/978-3-031-93634-0_4

appropriate and necessary. Good governance is therefore essential to the successful completion of the project.

This should not be a barrier to research. Although there are potentially many factors to consider, some basic principles and common frameworks do much of the heavy lifting. Much of the work is about making the time to think and then planning effectively for the project.

The aim of this chapter is to introduce key ideas in data governance (that is, ethics, data and people management, and disclosure control). It will not go into research methods, such as how to run successful interviews or how to run an RCT; these are covered in other parts of the book.

The Five Safes: A Structure for Planning

Good data governance is generally what you think when you have time to think. However, the way you think about it will affect the outcome, and different disciplines may have different views on what matters. We therefore start by considering *how* we should think about data governance and then introduce the framing we use in this chapter.

Data governance involves ethics, data management, disclosure control, people management, public engagement, and archiving policy. One common framework to manage these different interests is the Five Safes (Ritchie, 2017). This framework is used extensively in health and social science research in the UK, including the Ministry of Justice and the Department of Health.

The Five Safes breaks down governance into five separate but related areas (Table 4.1):

These dimensions of control are not rigid; they are designed to make planning easier by turning data governance into a series of smaller tasks.

Table 4.1 The five safes

Safe…	What questions are being asked?	Covers…
Projects	What are we aiming to do? What approvals do we need in place? How is the project going to run, and what happens at the end?	Broad purpose of project Ethical review Public engagement/ cost–benefit review Privacy impact assessments Post-project planning
Data	What data do we need to collect, and what will we be using for research?	De-identification and anonymisation
Setting	How are we going to store the data? How do we acquire, transfer, share it, and with whom?	Data flow diagram Data management plans Access controls
Outputs	How will we make sure there is no risk in outputs?	Output checks
People	What skills can we expect from our team to make this happen? Do we need to do training?	Training Job requirements

Safe Projects

'Safe projects' is about core project planning, and determining how you can embed positive practices throughout the project's journey. This section considers what an EpiCrim researcher should consider when scoping, applying for access, completing, and reporting on their project.

The initial planning phase is crucial to:

- clarify goals and planned activities
- anticipate problems
- provide accountability and transparency

A clear statement of what you are trying to achieve, why it is in the interests of society, and how you intend to manage the privacy risks to data subjects, is an excellent starting point. Once the set-up phase has been completed, the project will often diverge from initial plans; having that clear perspective on what you intend to achieve reduces the chance of missteps and mitigates the impact of unexpected problems.

The ethics application provides a solid foundation for a project governance record—one which captures and records changes in the project whilst providing the principal starting point for the project. You can follow the Five Safes structure if the ethics form does not have a clear or helpful format; this reduces the chance of missing something. The data governance plan format suggested at the end of this chapter may also be a useful starting point.

Ideally, the ethical review process should be a positive process for both reviewers and researchers that allows the project to become stronger. In practice, the application process can be poorly designed, burdensome and entrenched in bureaucracy; and it is often approached with fear or loathing by researchers. Nevertheless, try to approach it in a positive frame of mind because

(a) having a structure, any structure, really does helps planning
(b) the reviewers should have seen similar projects before and will be aware of potential pitfalls

The ethical review may be the one chance for an independent and knowledgeable 'critical friend' to have a detailed look at your project, so exploit the opportunity.

What to Include in Project Planning

As a starting checklist (which you will need for any ethical review, as well as your own project planning), you should have answers to each of these:

1. What is the public benefit, and is there a specific benefit to particular groups?
2. What are the privacy risks to the data subjects during data collection? How will they be managed?
3. What are the privacy risks to the data subjects from the storing and processing of their data? How will the risks be managed?
4. What other risks might participants face?
5. Will you obtain consent for data collection and use, or will some other gateway be more appropriate?

6. Who will have access to the data, and at what stages?
7. What happens to the data at the end of the project? Can it be re-used for other projects?

Forgetting to consider the last is frequent error. Research projects often focus on collecting the data and then realise at the project end that it can't be re-used, even in anonymous form, because consent wasn't obtained to deposit the data in an archive.

Point (2) is also often overlooked. When doing primary data collection, researchers tend to focus on getting the most valid data—but managing the privacy of your respondents is also important. Focus groups are particularly problematic because the purpose of the focus group (encouraging participants to speak freely and share with others) may be in direct conflict with the principle that participants should be prevented from incriminating themselves or others.

Informed Consent

All projects using PII require a demonstration of legality, legitimacy, and purpose before activities can commence. Informed consent is often treated as 'gold standard' for collecting primary data. It provides:

- Legal compliance with research and data usage
- Project legitimacy
- Protection for both researchers and participants
- A chance for you to state, clearly and in plain language, exactly how the project will be run

Incorporating informed consent into project planning involves assessing whether consent forms adequately cover any changes in the project plan or intended data usage. Informed consent holds particular significance for post-project activities, such as developing anonymised datasets for secondary analysis by other projects or creating teaching resources. To obtain informed consent, documents should

- Use clear and appropriate language in participant documentation; be sure to test its clarity and comprehensibility
- Provide a straightforward explanation of the project, data collection, usage, and storage plans
- Make explicit commitments regarding data protection and usage, such as data retention after the study's conclusion and any plans for data sharing
- Offer sufficient but manageable supporting information, which may include relevant links to distress and well-being organisations

Consent can be very useful when privacy constrains research unnecessarily. For example, consider a project which interviews a minister for prison policy. Quotes from that person may be particularly valuable if it can be reported who made the comments. Getting consent to use an identified quote may be much more effective than trying to anonymise the quote but keep it informative.

Other Legal Gateways: Administrative and Secondary Data

Informed consent is not the only gateway. It may not always be appropriate or achievable, especially within EpiCrim. When acquiring administrative data for research (for example, from prison data) consent is normally not possible. Within the UK legal framework, there is almost always a lawful basis for acquiring data for research, but it may vary depending on the type of data, the organisation that holds the data, and how you plan to acquire, treat, use and archive the data. If the data you wish to use has been used before, the chances are that the same procedures can be re-used. Even if this is the first research use of some data, start negotiations with the assumption that the data *can* be used for research, and the question is *how* to make it usable. This will be more effective if you can identify the value to the data provider—so make sure you are clear about the benefits of the research.

When secondary data (i.e. already collected and prepared for research) is being used, the organisation providing the data (for example, the

UK Data Archive) will normally have set up the appropriate approval processes. Make sure you comply with those procedures—an external organisation will have little sympathy with you if you try bending the rules. Your ethics board may still require you to inform them, so check your organisation's procedures.

Ethical Considerations: Beyond Consent

When engaging with vulnerable individuals facing complexities like active psychosis, paranoia, or short-term memory loss, obtaining written informed consent may not always be straightforward; but other gateways are not magic bullets. Legal gateways for research almost always require you to demonstrate that the research is ethically justified. The researcher responsible for data collection must exercise professional judgement to determine whether participation is in the participant's best interest or beneficial at that specific moment.

It is difficult working within grey areas, as often we come across scenarios and situations of which we had not planned for and there is no clear answer. We are required to make a judgement. In such cases, we need to go back to first principles to help us navigate our behaviours.

A common set of principles used is the Belmont principles (DHHS, 1979) which outlines the following criteria for research:

1. Respecting individuals involves safeguarding their autonomy and treating them with courtesy and respect
2. Beneficence dictates a commitment to minimising harm and maximising benefits for both the research and participant.
3. Justice requires fair and equitable procedures, ensuring the reasonable distribution of costs and benefits amongst participants.

Safe Data

When we think of data types, we tend to focus on how the data is structured; for example, is it qualitative or quantitative, small or large scale, administrative or survey? However, in this section we are going to think of data in terms of how identifiable the data is (Table 4.2).

Identified Data

Identified data is typically a product of the data acquisition stage of a research project. For quantitative analysis, de-identifying data is normally straightforward. Direct identifiers such as name are unlikely to have research value and so can be replaced by a non-informative index.[2]

For qualitative data where you want to retain some information, you may want to indicate an important characteristic of the data subject in the index 'Participant M(ale)3 stated…'. It is possible that you are not

Table 4.2 Types of personal data and how it links to EpiCrim

Type	Meaning	EpiCrim example
Identified	Data contains information allowing the data subject to be directly identified, such as name and address, NHS number, or court record number	Official court records including name, address, felony, and official record
De-identified	No piece of information on its own directly identifies the person, but combinations of data, perhaps with other information, could reasonably lead to re-identification	Court records with name and record number converted to random index, but containing participant's age, gender, conviction, court district, and month of conviction
Anonymous	No reasonable likelihood of someone being able to re-identify this person	Court records with age and gender, felony and sentence presented in broad categories, no court details

[2] If the respondent is Mr Bruce Dickinson of 22 Acacia Avenue BS11 1QY then "participant 07" is non-informative, "patient BD.BS11" is not.

able to redact effectively without losing much of the data detail; in this case, the controls on settings and people will be the key guarantees of data security. This is a key lesson of the Five Safes approach: you should aim to reduce unnecessary identifiers, but you do *not* have to redact relevant research information if you can manage it effectively in other ways (for example, through consent to name interviewees).

You may need to retain direct identifiers so you can link to the original participants—for example, for quality control, or if data is coming from multiple sources and needs to be matched. Another case is where you need to re-contact the participant, such as in a longitudinal study. Finally, if you have given participants an opportunity to withdraw from the study, you need to retain the contact information for as long as the right-to-withdraw lasts. Keep this information separate from the research data and use a lookup file to link the index with the direct identifiers. See Fig. 4.1.

In general, try to avoid collecting identifiers. For example, if running an online survey, do not ask for participant's name or email unless essential—if you do, your data management becomes much harder. Similarly, if writing up notes from an interview, use a synonym to reference the interview.

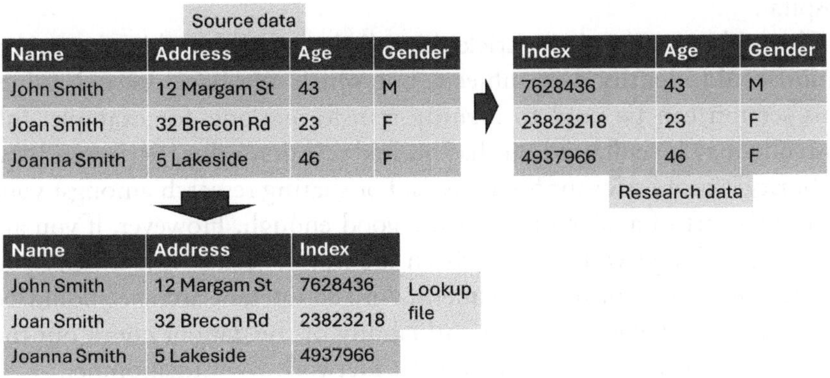

Fig. 4.1 Separating source data into research data and lookup files

De-Identified Data

Your data may not have direct identifiers, but it might include information which allows a person to be identified by combing multiple variables. Consider:

- what combinations of variables are likely to be unique in population/ in datasets? (for example, postcode + age + gender; court appearance date + offence + sentence; date of birth + treatment + hospital)
- Are some variables particularly problematic? If so, are they really needed (is date of birth needed, or is age in years good enough?)
- Is it likely someone could be known to be part of the data? (for example, people observed going into the interview room)

We developed the following template for researchers to help them classify outputs—see Fig. 4.2, which has been completed for an imaginary project studying road traffic collisions:

The first section lists the identifiers—these should not be in the research dataset but may need to be retained for management purposes. The third section identifies variables of research interest but with no meaningful identification; for example, type of road, length of stay in hospital.

The middle section is the tricky bit—listing variables which in combination could identify data subjects, but which also have research value. This section can be used to identify transformations: for example, full postcode may be collected but has limited research value, whereas a local authority is more relevant for analysis. For sharing research amongst your team, this sort of analysis is probably good enough. However, if you are planning to lodge your data with an archive or share with others, you should consider a formal assessment. Any competent archive should be able to provide advice on the identifiability of the data or check out the guidance from the UK Anonymisation Network www.ukanon.net.

Variable	Sensitivity	Uniqueness / distinctiveness	Needed for: Participant management	Linking	Analysis
Direct identifiers					
Name	Low	Almost unique	Yes	No linking	No
Health service number	High	Unique	Yes	No linking	No
Indirect identifiers					
Date of birth	High	Rare in sample, common in population	Yes		Yes
Postcode (approx. 40 people)	Low	Rare in sample, Rare in population	Yes		No
Local authority district (approx. 4000 people)	Low	Repeated in sample, common in population	No		Yes
Ethnicity	Medium	Repeated in sample, common in population	No		Yes
Age	Low	Common in sample	Yes		Yes
Gender (M/F)	Low	Very common in sample	Yes		Yes
Registered patient at hospital	High	Very common in sample, rare in population	No		Yes
Non-identifiers					
Weather conditions at time of RTC	Low	n/a	No	No	Yes
Road type	Low	n/a	No	No	Yes
Injury	High	n/a	No	No	Yes
Length of stay in hospital					
...et cetera					

Identifying combinations of indirect identifiers

Almost certainly unique for participants and in the population:

- Date of birth, postcode, gender
- Date of birth, postcode, registered patient

Likely to be unique in the sample and population

- Age, postcode, gender
- Age, postcode, ethnicity
- Date of birth, local authority, gender, ethnicity, registered patient

Potentially unique in sample, not in population

- Age, local authority, gender, ethnicity
- Age, local authority, registered patient, gender, ethnicity

Identifiers; Remove

Indirect identifiers; Assess

Non-identifiers; Keep

Assessment

Fig. 4.2 Template for understanding data risk

Anonymous and Public Domain Data

If the data are truly anonymous, then many of your problems do go away. This does not mean no responsibilities—there may be ethical reasons for managing or restricting access, or your informed consent may not allow unrestricted re-use of the data. Data in the public domain is not a free-for-all. There may be ethical or commercial factors to consider, and there are a few (obscure) legal factors which might be important—for example, combining publicly available data into an easily accessible form for mass analysis can create a new PII dataset. As for anonymised data, don't assume that it's fine to share—get a second opinion before doing so.

Special Category Data

The GDPR (and local implementations, such as the UK Data Protection Act 2018) specify certain 'special category' data to which particular care should be applied. These are

- personal data revealing racial or ethnic origin;
- personal data revealing political opinions;
- personal data revealing religious or philosophical beliefs;
- personal data revealing trade union membership;
- genetic data;
- biometric data (where used for identification purposes);
- data concerning health;
- data concerning a person's sex life; and
- data concerning a person's sexual orientation.

EpiCrim data is likely to be in one or more of these categories. In theory, this means you should be able to show that you meet both the general conditions for processing data, and additional conditions for processing special category data. From a research perspective, it is not clear how useful this is in practice. Getting informed consent, or approval for processing unconsented data for research purposes in the public interest, should cover both regular and special category data. Your guiding principle should be 'don't let the data be shared with anyone who shouldn't have access' rather than trying to fine tune access dependent on specific variables. Full details on processing special category data is in the ICO guidance https://ico.org.uk/for-organisations/uk-gdpr-guidance-and-resources/lawful-basis/a-guide-to-lawful-basis/.

Safe Settings

Technical storage of the data needs to address two problems:

- Is the data appropriately secure for the level of risk in the data?
- Can the researchers use the data effectively?

The first point is obvious, but the second also matters. If researchers are required to use an awkward technical solution, they will often find ways around your management strategy (such as emailing the data to themselves to work on at home) so this is a significant risk. Luckily, modern universities provide adequate and usable storage for most research needs. Secured servers with backups allow researchers to work easily in a restricted environment, and systems such as Microsoft OneDrive allow researchers to manage access directly irrespective of physical location. However, make that you are working in an appropriate environment; for example, not in a public space like a café, and not using public Wi-Fi.

Ensure that shared folder access is limited only to those on the project team. This is one of the easiest things to do to protect your data, but also easily forgotten as team members join and leave. If you need to store identifiers, make sure that these are kept in secure folders separate from the research dataset, and only allow access to the subset *within* your project team who absolutely must have this information.

A helpful way to visualise the process is to do a **data flow diagram**. For example, Fig. 4.3 shows a very simple example of how contact data from a summer school and a survey were collected and transformed into an opt-in mailing list and a dataset for analysis:

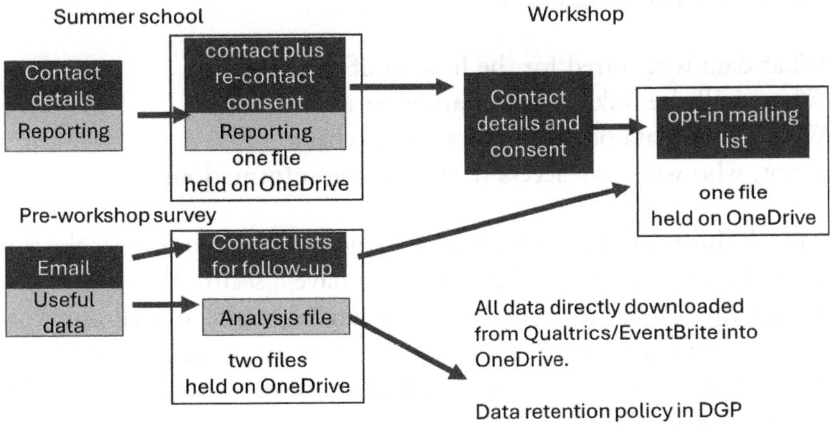

Fig. 4.3 Example data flow diagram

This simple example merely lists the type of data and where it is held. For a real research project, the diagram should show each step of the data flows including, for each stage

- Where is the data stored?
- what format will the data be held in (for example collected as an audio file, then transcribed into Word).
- how does data move from one stage to the next?
- where are identifiers removed?
- where does linking happen?
- which, if any, of these are long-term storage solutions?

For external and internal team members accessing the database:

- why do they need access to the data?
- what can they use that data for?
- who would be aware if data was improperly accessed or used?
- will the researchers use the secure environment?
- what security measures will be in place in that research environment?
- what personal data will be included in that database?

For data which is being linked:

- What data is required for the linking of the data?
- Where will the linking information be stored?
- Will linking data be accessible to researchers?
- If not, who will have access to the linking information?

Listing all this information for a small project is likely to be over the top, because the answer is very likely to be 'we have a secure University drive that only the project team has access to, and we carry out all our work there'. However, as a project grows, checklists and diagrams will be an important part of understanding your technical risks and demonstrating how you manage them.

If you have particularly sensitive data, you may need to use a secure research facility ('trusted research environment' or TRE), such as UK Data Archive's SecureLab. SAIL at Swansea University runs over twenty dedicated TREs for different projects. TREs are best practice for managing secure research access to the most sensitive data.

Safe People

Researchers generally are well-intentioned, clever people; but they are also liable to be lazy; forgetful; set in their ways; over-confident in own trustworthiness; and good at side-stepping processes they dislike. In other words, human. It is important to design processes for humans. For example, if researchers are required to use a server which doesn't have full functionality, then researchers will end up downloading files to work offline, *and* the project manager loses credibility.

Hence, best practice in data governance training focuses on building a data community, where team members feel valued and trusted, and understand their role in data governance. Developing a no-blame culture for identifying mistakes or poor practices is an important part of this process. This is harder work than simply telling project members what they need to do, but there is ample evidence now that encouraging positive behaviours is far more effective in the long run for ensuring good data governance. This is a research topic in itself, but Green and Ritchie (2023) provide an overview.

Safe Outputs

Completing ethics and ensuring that only named individuals have access to raw data isn't enough to fully protect privacy. The publication of research results can lead to unintended consequences, especially when derived from very small, specific populations or individuals (such as those studied in EpiCrim). An inadvertent disclosure occurs when a reader of the research sees that some confidential information has been revealed. We also need to consider the possibility that an 'intruder' actively attempts to obtain specific information (such as locating and identifying a particular prisoner).

This is disclosure control. It is rarely taught in research methods, but a basic understanding is essential when working with confidential data. You should ensure that at least one person on your team is familiar with these concepts and consult them for a second opinion before releasing outputs from confidential data. There are training courses and materials for statistical disclosure control; see www.saferesearchertraining.org. Unfortunately, there is very little material or training for qualitative outputs other than learning on the job.

Statistical Disclosure Control (SDC) in Quantitative Data

Imagine an RCT exploring the impact of structured high intensity exercise sessions on mental wellbeing in long-term male inmates across three different prisons. Two of the published tables are Tables 4.3 and 4.4.

What happens if we were to begin to combine data across the tables? Table 4.4 says that there are only 3 people in Prison A. The 'N/A' suggests

Table 4.3 Descriptive statistics across groups

Condition	Mean Age	Min	Max	Std	Mean sentence (excl. whole life sentences)	Min	Max	Std	Whole life sentences
Control	51.02	28	72	13.05	17.24	12	30	6.01	2
Treatment	51.58	23	71	12.92	18.44	12	30	6.62	1

Table 4.4 Descriptive statistics across prisons and groups

	Prison A N = 3		Prison B N = 5		Prison C N = 30	
	Age	Length of sentence	Age	Length of sentence	Age	Length of sentence
Control group	43	N/A	51.5	14.50	52.1	17.60
Treatment group	23	N/A	60	23.00	51.8	17.53

Table 4.5 Descriptive statistics across prisons and groups

	Prison A N = 3		Prison B N = 5		Prison C N = 30	
	Age	Length of sentence	Age	Length of sentence	Age	Length of sentence
Control group	43	N/A	51.5	14.50	52.1	17.60
Treatment group	23	N/A	60	23.00	51.8	17.53

that there is a structural reason sentence length can't be calculated; it is reasonable to assume (and easily checked) that Prison A exclusively holds the whole lifers. But Table 4.3 shows that there are 3 prisoners who have a whole life sentence, 2 in the control group, 1 in the treatment group (Table 4.5). So Table 4.4 is now.

Table 4.6 Descriptice statistics across prisons and groups with additional information

	Prison A N = 3		Prison B N = 5		Prison C N = 30	
	Age	Length of sentence	Age	Length of sentence	Age	Length of sentence
Control group	43 N = = 2	N/A Whole life	51.5	14.50	52.1	17.60
Treatment group	23 N = = 1	N/A Whole life	60	23.00	51.8	17.53

The age of the single individual in Prison A treatment group is now revealed to everyone. In addition, the age of the Prison A inmates in the control group is revealed to each of them; for example, if one inmate is aged 27, he knows that the other is aged 59 (43 × 2–27), and vice versa. This is why three is given in all the textbooks as the **minimum frequency** for a 'safe' count.

Having calculated Prison A groups, we can fill in other information using basic maths. We can even use information such as the average length of sentence reported in Table 4.3, compare it with the average length of sentence in each prison and use this to calculate the split of participants (Table 4.7).

If one had additional information (for example, knowing that the maximum sentence of 30 years listed in Table 4.1 is associated with one of the treatment group in Prison B), then more information could be extracted and the identity of participants revealed.

This is a concern for EpiCrim, because characteristics such as age, gender and sentence length may be publicly recorded. Imagine that 18 months ago an infamous murderer received a whole life tariff at the age of 21. His age and his crimes made him of commercial interest to the newspapers, who reported that he was the first person under 30 in 15 years to be given a whole life tariff (Table 4.6). Is he in the treatment group, the control group, or neither?

Finally, what can we tell from Table 4.8?

Table 4.7 Prisons B and C analysed

	Prison A N = 3		Prison B N = 5		Prison C N = 30		Total (A + B + C) N = 38
	Age	Length of sentence	Age	Length of sentence	Age	Length of sentence	
Control group N = 19	43 N = 2	N/A	51.5 N = 2	14.50	52.1 N = 15	17.60	Control group (A + B + C) N = 19 Average sentence = 17.24 (from Table 4.1)
Treatment group N = 19	23 N = 1	N/A	60 N = 3	23.00	51.8 N = 15	17.53	Treatment group (A + B + C) N = 19 Average sentence = 18.44 (from Table 4.1)

Table 4.8 Other health conditions present in participants

Other health conditions present (% diagnosed in group participants)	Control Group N = 19 (%)	Treatment Group N = 19 (%)
Depression and Anxiety	100	100
HIV	0	5
Schizoaffective disorder	20	10
Hypertension	45	55
Diabetes type 2	55	55
Restless legs syndrome	100	55

100% of all participants have been diagnosed with depression and anxiety; therefore, if you know any participant in the study, you now know this about them. This is 'group disclosure' or 'class disclosure': just belonging to a particular group/ class allows you to learn something about that person. If you know someone in the control group, you know they have been diagnosed with 'restless legs syndrome', but not HIV. Finally, the one person (5% × 19) HIV-positive in the treatment group now knows that no-one else is HIV-positive.

Analytical results (such regression models or ANOVA) do not generally present disclosure risks. The problematic results are always in simple statistics. As general rules

- have at least three or more observations underlying any statistic
- be careful where a statistic can be applied to everyone in a group (i.e. 100% or 0% of the group have some characteristic)
- avoid very skewed distributions, or outliers in graphs

Broadly speaking, there are three solutions to problematic results

- Suppress the numbers (adjust any totals after suppression)
- Add uncertainty to the numbers, for example by rounding
- Re-design the statistics to present the information in another way

There is a large literature on this, but see

- Lowthian and Ritchie (2017) for a basic introduction
- Green and Ritchie (2021) for a summary of protection measures

- Griffiths et al. (2019) for a detailed set of examples
- SACRO (2023) for a fully comprehensive guide

Qualitative Data

By its nature, qualitative data focuses on individual experience rather than average effects, and so disclosure is much more likely than in quantitative data. Unfortunately the literature in this area focuses on providing generic guidance surrounding data collection and ethics, and there is little structured guidance for ensuring outputs are not disclosive.

Consider the following quote taken from a (fictional) project report

> "... they (other residents) ran the prison, Spice was brought through the post it was sprayed onto the baking paper catering supplies. The head chef was part of it, he was in deep so many staff members were in debt it was just us (the residents) ..." Cat C Inmate, HMP Westland

The quote doesn't name names, but it names the prison and a unique role there; assuming the project gives some idea of the time period covered by the report, this is directly and unambiguously identifying an individual.

The US Census Bureau has recently introduced a checklist and guiding principles to ensure documents are de-identified. The recommended steps/checks include:

- Removing names and locations
- Eliminating dates
- Omitting proper nouns
- Providing descriptive demographics only if they cannot be linked with other information to uniquely identify participants
- Eliminating all data that could potentially be matched with publicly available databases
- Excluding photos, videos, and voice recordings
- Using direct quotes only if they do not contain unique information

In cases involving unusual quotations, search engines can be employed to verify the quote's authenticity and potential linkage to personal information elsewhere.

An example of transforming a (fictional) quote:

> Original: "I had nowhere to go and I had just been diagnosed as HIV positive. My world was spiralling, I was due to be released originally I was going to stay with my aunt in St Pauls, but on release I went and nicked a Porsche 911 and got in a police car chase across Bristol. I ended up back in custody that night." Cat A Inmate, HMP Westland
> Transformed: "I had nowhere to go, and I had just been diagnosed as HIV positive. My world was spiralling, I was due to be released originally, I was going to stay with family, but on release I went and nicked a car. I ended up back in custody that night." Cat A inmate, Prison 3

Sharing the findings or write-up with participants serves to demonstrate how quotes are being used and interpreted by researchers. While this may not always be feasible, especially with anonymous quotes, an alternative approach is to share the initial report draft with contributors and invite them to raise any concerns with the research team. Note however, that participants may not be the best judge of what is 'identifiable'—your judgement is what matters.

In some cases, you may want to use named quotes; for example, the view of a prison governor is important because she is the prison governor. In these cases, get consent (ideally at the data collection stage, retrospectively if you must), but also make sure that the participants are content to be associated with the quote.

Post-Project Blues

One area often forgotten in project planning is what will happen to the data post-project. If your data turns out to be extremely valuable, can you make it available to others? Not unless it was in your consent form (for consented data), or in the agreement with the data providers (for other data). It may be possible to contact the data provider to change the terms of access, but for primary data collection, re-contacting data subjects to ask for a change of use is both unethical and a poor research outcome. This is why informed consent is a double-edged sword: get it right and the world is your friend; get it wrong, and you can end up severely hampering your research.

The other frequent pitfall is not knowing what kind of data you will be archiving. Consent forms often state that only anonymous data will be made available, whereas in fact the research teams plans to deposit de-identified data. This is not allowed.

So: make sure that your original proposals include a plan for what happens at the end of the project; and that any commitments you make are consistent with that long-term plan. Be particularly clear whether any archiving includes identifiable or anonymous data, and who can have access to that data.

Constructing Data Governance Plans

You may find it helpful to construct a data governance plan. This covers similar ground to the ethical application, but it is wider. Nevertheless, re-use as much material as possible from other documents you are required to produce—as well as saving you time, this ensures consistency across different processes.

We developed a template for our data governance courses which has been proved relatively successful for researcher to use and adapt. It consists of six sections:

1. Description of the project: what is it about, type of data, public benefit, potential risks
2. Relevant documents and where to find them: ethics approval, data management plan, university data security policy, and so on
3. Inherent data risk assessment—(see Fig. 4.2)
4. Data flow diagram
5. Risk-response matrix
6. Table of actions

The risk-response matrix aims to identify all reasonable risks associated with the project, and list the response: something we have done, something we plan to do, something we are not going to deal with because we feel it does not warrant a response. Figure 4.4 gives an example.

The aim is to list as many potential risks as possible and ensure that they are dealt with. This is best done as a group exercise within the project team; otherwise, the project manager tends to list things they

Issue	Risk	Response
Projects		
Ethics	Consent not informed	Ethics Committee check and approve
	Consent not comprehensive	Ethics Committee check and approve
	Consent limits range of feasible research too much	Ethics Committee check and approve
	Study participants may want to know findings of tests if negative	Participant information sheet states exactly what information will be given back to participants; ethics Committee check and approve
	Participants want to withdraw but cannot	Participant information sheet states exactly when participants can withdraw data; ethics Committee check and approve Data management plan needs to ensure this is feasible
Public benefit/engagement	Project cannot start/ends early because of lack of public support	Ensure public engagement strategy is in place
	No data contributions as project team not seen as trustworthy	Get buy-in from [respected people/organisation] and quote this and ethics approval on all documents for interviewees
Data governance	No DG as no responsible person	X to have formal responsibility for planning reviewing reporting on DG
Post project	Consent doesn't all post-project sharing or archiving	Ethics Committee check and approve
People		
Data collectors	Collectors may recognise people in the dataset	Training in good data practices – to be set up
	Collectors may talk about the people they collected data	Training in good data practices – to be set up

Fig. 4.4 Example risk-response matrix

Table 4.9 Example table of actions

Control	Action needed	Response
Projects	Need long-term storage option	X to confirm storage plans before October 2023
People	Training on good practice for confidential data—for researchers	To be done by dd.mm
	Training on good practice for confidential data—for data collectors	To be done by dd.mm

have already dealt with. You may also find it useful to have a facilitator familiar with data governance to prompt queries.

Finally, you should have a table of actions for dealing with the issues raised in the risk-response matrix. This is where you list what needs to be done, by whom, by when (Table 4.9):

This is where your data governance plan changes from being an initial proposal, to a living document that you need to review and update. The good news is, everything you tick off is another problem addressed.

Ready to Go?

Data governance is a large topic, with specialists in each area. This chapter has covered much of the ground at a high level, identifying broad areas of good practice, and some specific advice where experience shows researchers are most likely to make mistakes.

In practice, data governance is less complicated than sometimes presented. With the exception of 'safe outputs', much of the material in this chapter should be familiar. The key elements of successful data governance are:

- Good advance planning, with a structure that makes sense to you
- Use mandatory requirements (such as ethical review forms) positively to go through potential issues
- Distinguish between what could possibly go wrong and what may reasonably go wrong; address the latter; don't fret about the former

- Focus on 'where do we want to be' and work out how to get there, rather than focusing on what is an isn't possible/allowable; in other words, make ethics your guide
- Build a positive, collaborative, trusting and trustworthy team

Templates and examples of completed data governance plans can be found at http://www.saferesearchertraining.org/data_governance/templates.

References

DHHS. (1979). *The Belmont report: Ethical principles and guidelines for the protection of human subjects of research.* U.S. Department of Health and Human Services: National Commission for the Protection of Human Subjects of Biomedical and Behavioral Research. https://www.hhs.gov/ohrp/regulations-and-policy/belmont-report/read-the-belmont-report/index.html. Accessed February 23, 2025.

Green, E., & Ritchie, F. (2021). Statistical disclosure control for HESA: Part 1: Review of SDC theory. *Higher Education Statistics Agency (HESA).* https://uwe-repository.worktribe.com/output/10621148/. Accessed February 23, 2025.

Green, E., & Ritchie, F. (2023). Using pedagogical and psychological insights to train analysts using confidential data. *Journal of Privacy and Confidentiality, 13*(2). https://doi.org/10.29012/jpc.842

Griffiths, E., Greci, C., Kortrotsios, Y., Parker, S., Scott, J., Welpton, R., Wolters, A., & Woods, C. (2019). *Handbook on statistical disclosure control for outputs. Safe data access professionals working group.* https://doi.org/10.6084/m9.figshare.9958520. Accessed February 23, 2025.

Lowthian, P., & Ritchie, F. (2017). *Ensuring the confidentiality of statistical outputs from the ADRN.* Report for ADRN. https://uwe-repository.worktribe.com/output/888435. Accessed February 23, 2025.

Ritchie, F. (2017, September) The "Five Safes": A framework for planning, designing and evaluating data access solutions. *Data for Policy 2017*. https://doi.org/10.5281/zenodo.897821. Accessed February 23, 2025.

SACRO. (2023). *SACRO guide to statistical output checking*. https://doi.org/10.5281/zenodo.10054629. Accessed February 23, 2025.

Part II

Prevention

5

Examining the Role of Online Communities in the Prevention of Child Sexual Abuse

Nick Addis, Ella Rees, Ian Johnson, Phil Legg, and Maggie Brennan

Introduction

In 2024, the Internet Watch Foundation (IWF) confirmed the presence of 291,273 webpages containing child sexual abuse (CSA) imagery, links to imagery, or the advertising of this (a 5% increase from 2023; IWF, 2025a). This represents the largest number of CSA webpages the IWF has found in its 29-year history, as well as an 830% increase in online child sexual abuse (OCSA) imagery since IWF began to proactively hunt CSA in 2014 (IWF, 2025a). Moreover, each individual website hosting such content could contain hundreds or thousands of CSA images/videos

N. Addis (✉) · E. Rees · I. Johnson · P. Legg
University of the West of England, Bristol, UK
e-mail: Nick.Addis@uwe.ac.uk

E. Rees
e-mail: Ella.Rees@uwe.ac.uk

I. Johnson
e-mail: Ian.Johnson@uwe.ac.uk

K. McCartan et al. (eds.), *Developing and Implementing a Public Health and Criminological Approach to Tackling Sexual Abuse*, Palgrave Studies in Risk, Crime and Society, https://doi.org/10.1007/978-3-031-93634-0_5

(IWF, 2023). Childlight, the Global Child Safety Institute at the University of Edinburgh identified that in the last 12 months, over 300 million children under the age of 18 had been affected by online child sexual exploitation and abuse, and 1 in 8 children had experienced solicitation online, and non-consensual taking, sharing and/or exposure to sexual images and videos (Childlight, 2024). As such, this provides an initial indication as to the scale of this issue. Moreover, WeProtect Global Alliance estimate that the level of reported child sexual abuse material (CSAM) has risen by 87% since 2019 (WeProtect Global Alliance, 2023), indicating the level of growth in this area.

To help frame these crimes, the term, 'Online Child Sexual Abuse and Exploitation' can be used to cover a number of different offences, including online grooming; live streaming; online coercion and blackmail; and the possession, production, and sharing of indecent and prohibited images and videos of children (Child Exploitation and Online Protection, 2024). Child sexual exploitation (CSE) is a form of CSA, i.e. where an individual or group takes advantage of an imbalance of power to coerce, manipulate or deceive a child or young person under the age of 18 into sexual activity (Child Exploitation and Online Protection, 2024). However, for the purposes of this chapter, focus will be upon collective efforts to fight these crimes more broadly, i.e. through the role of organisations acting as capable guardians, and restricting access to victims, rather than considering responses for CSA and CSE separately.

Instances of OCSA and exploitation are facilitated through online communities accessible via the surface web (i.e. social media platforms such as Facebook, X (formerly Twitter), Instagram, TikTok, as well as online gaming communities). Indeed, there is a body of work exploring the use of social media platforms by perpetrators to engage in OCSA (Ali et al., 2023; Weingraber et al., 2020). Though it is known sexual harms

P. Legg
e-mail: Phil.Legg@uwe.ac.uk

M. Brennan
Dublin City University, Dublin, Ireland
e-mail: Maggie.Brennan@dcu.ie

also occur across the video game, streaming, and esports communities, research into abuse across these domains remains in its relative infancy (Merry & Whitfield, 2024). For organisations to effectively tackle the proliferation of OCSA across their platforms, it remains imperative that they implement a range of measures, across varying points of intervention. This chapter focuses on the role played by online communities, i.e. social media platforms, technology companies, gaming organisations and the charity sector, in preventing OCSA.

Alignment with the Epidemiological Criminology Perspective

The scale and growing nature of this problem necessitates the need for this to be treated as a global public health issue in urgent need of a wider response (Data Driven Innovation, 2024). As noted by Paul Stanfield, CEO of Childlight Global Child Safety Institute (and former senior officer in the National Crime Agency and former Interpol Director), 'This is a global health pandemic that has remained hidden for far too long. It occurs in every country; it's growing exponentially and it requires a global response. We need to act urgently and treat it as a public health issue that can be prevented.' (Stanfield, cited in Data Driven Innovation, 2024).

The call for OCSA to be viewed as a global public health issue aligns with the Epidemiological Criminology (Epi-Crim) focus. Lanier (2010) notes how Epi-Crim covers, '…the study of anything that affects the health of a society…crime, flu epidemics, global warming, human trafficking, substance abuse, terrorism or HIV/AIDS' (Lanier, 2010, p. 72). To tackle any such issue requires a coordinated and collaborative response, across differing levels of geographical focus. OCSA is no exception. The nature of this problem clearly lends itself to the consideration of responses at varying geographical scales; specifically, those at the macro- (societal), meso- (community), and micro- (individual/interpersonal) levels. Responses at the macro-level may be those formed by national governments, or by technology companies themselves; meso-level responses may include those by local communities, local councils, and school interventions; with micro-level responses potentially by friends, parents or caregivers, or children themselves.

The current chapter will focus largely on macro-level responses; specifically, technology companies that host online communities in which OCSA takes place. In particular, the chapter will explore a range of responses provided by social media or gaming platforms to tackle the torrent of OCSA experienced in recent years, before considering some of the challenges faced in enacting such initiatives and thinking about areas worthy of future attention. However, before considering possible responses, the chapter will consider the legislative backdrop within which such responses are framed, as this forms a key driver for technology organisations to act in the fight against OCSA.

Legislative Framework: The Online Safety Act 2023

The Online Safety Act 2023 is a new set of legislation protecting children and adults, placing a range of responsibilities on social media organisations, holding them accountable for users' safety on their sites (Gov.uk, 2025a). The Act holds technology companies to account for any content hosted on their platforms, ensuring such organisations take action to prevent the proliferation of OCSA (Gov.uk, 2025a). These measures include removing illegal content or preventing it from appearing initially, providing parents and young people with mechanisms to highlight issues as they arise, preventing children from being able to access dangerous/age-inappropriate content, ensuring greater transparency amongst organisations of the risks to children on their platforms, and enacting age limits and age-checking measures on sites where harmful content can be hosted (Gov.uk, 2023a).

As the regulator for UK online safety, Ofcom must ensure platforms protect their users, and will have powers to take action against companies not adhering to these duties. This includes platforms that are based overseas where there are a significant number of UK users, platforms where

UK users present as a target market, or where platforms hosting content may present a significant risk of harm to the UK public (Gov.uk, 2025a).

The Rt Hon Peter Kyle MP (Secretary of State for Department for Science, Innovation and Technology) set out the Government's strategic priorities for online safety (Gov.uk, 2025b); the first of which being to, 'Embed safety by design', pushing the responsibility for online safety onto organisations that host online content, limiting the risk of harm posed to users. This includes the use of age-assurance (and other existing) technologies, to ensure children are unable to access harmful content on their platforms, and ensure that online services accessed are age-appropriate (Gov.uk, 2025b).

The drive to ensure online platforms are 'safe by design' aligns closely with the crime prevention literature; specifically, Routine Activity Theory (Cohen & Felson, 1979). According to Routine Activity Theory, for a crime to occur, three elements are required to be present: a motivated offender, a suitable target, and a lack of capable guardian (Cohen & Felson, 1979). In the fight against OCSA, technology companies typically play a key role as capable guardian figures, essentially limiting access for motivated offenders to suitable targets. However, to further understand the role of such capable guardians, it is important to define the nature of online communities, to establish the interplay between capable guardians and members of such online communities in the fight against OCSA.

Understanding Online Communities

The definition of online communities offered by the NSPCC may be particularly pertinent here: '*Online communities are groups of people that come together in a virtual environment*' (NSPCC, 2024). Thus, in terms of what can be enacted within such online communities in the fight against preventing OCSA, it can be considered that it is those who *occupy* such online spaces, alongside the organisations that host such spaces, as well as other organisations dedicated specifically to child safety, who are the key players (and potential capable guardians) in the fight against OCSA. Such organisations dedicated to online child safety include the

Internet Watch Foundation,[1] WeProtect Global Alliance,[2] the National Center for Missing and Exploited Children,[3] The National Society for the Prevention of Cruelty to Children (or NSPCC[4]), and the Technology Coalition.[5] As such, collaboration is at the heart of efforts to tackle the proliferation of OCSA activity.

Approaches Used to Tackle Online Child Sexual Abuse

The Role of Collaboration

The ethos of collaboration is shared by several technology organisations across social media and gaming platforms. For example, Microsoft (whose portfolio includes Xbox gaming studios), acknowledge the importance of collaboration, through making photo-matching technology, i.e. PhotoDNA (which helps identify copies of known abusive material to prevent people sharing these), freely available to qualified organisations (Microsoft, 2025a). PhotoDNA works by creating a

[1] The Internet Watch Foundation (IWF) are an independent, non-profit charitable organisation working in partnership with a range of other organisations/groups from the private, public and NGO sectors to minimise, disrupt and stop the availability of child sexual abuse images and videos hosted anywhere in the world, and non-photographic child sexual abuse images hosted in the UK (IWF, 2025b). Such organisations and groups include internet and technology industries, global law enforcement, governments, the education sector, charities and non-profit organisations across the world, and the general public (IWF, 2025b).

[2] WeProtect Global Alliance is a global movement dedicated to ending the online sexual exploitation and abuse of children. They bring together governments, private sector, civil society, and international organisations to create a safer digital world where every child can thrive (We Protect Global Alliance, 2025).

[3] The National Center for Missing and Exploited Children (NCMEC) is a non-profit organisation that works to help find missing children, reduce child sexual exploitation, and prevent child victimization (NCMEC, 2025a).

[4] The NSPCC is a national charity organisation who conduct a wide range of work to prevent child abuse and neglect (NSPCC, 2021).

[5] The Technology Coalition is an alliance of global technological organisations working together to address child sexual exploitation and abuse online (Technology Coalition, 2025).

unique digital signature (or 'hash'), which is then tested against signatures of other photos to identify replicas of the same image (Microsoft, 2025b).

TikTok similarly use multiple technologies, including their own, as well as hash-matching software such as Microsoft's PhotoDNA, Google's Content Safety API, and YouTube's CSAI Match. Alongside partners, TikTok have developed 'hash databases', which catalogue unique digital codes associated with known CSAM. If users upload material matching a digital code from TikTok's database, that content would be taken down, reported to the National Center for Missing and Exploited Children, and to law enforcement authorities, with any violating accounts subsequently banned (TikTok, 2025).

Sony Interactive Entertainment (SIE), who run the PlayStation Network,[6] utilise a combination of automated content detection tools, as well as human moderator teams to review reports of inappropriate content or misconduct. Such automated tools also make use of hash-matching software, with possible matches removed or sent to human moderation teams for further review (Sony Interactive Entertainment, 2025b).

A further illustration of collaboration and the sharing of technology across organisations can be seen through the 'Lantern' programme. The Lantern Programme is an innovative, cross-platform initiative that brings together social media platforms and other multinational technology organisations to share 'signals' about activity in breach of their policies against CSE. Signals may include details linked to violating accounts, such as e-mails, usernames or keywords used. Whilst in themselves signals do not provide *proof* of CSA activity, they can offer hints or indicators worthy of further investigation, to help reveal 'real-time' threats to children's safety (Technology Coalition, 2023). The Lantern Project launched with an initial group of companies joining the first phase, including Discord, Google, Mega, Meta (who own Facebook, Instagram, and WhatsApp), Quora, Roblox, Snap, and Twitch (Technology Coalition, 2023).

[6] Sony's online platform where users can play games, connect with other users, stream video content, purchase/download content (Sony Interactive Entertainment, 2025a).

What is also key to recognise is that collaboration is not simply restricted to social media platforms themselves. For example, Yoti, a global digital identity and biometric technology company, provide age-verification services for social media platforms (Meta, 2022; Yoti, 2021). The IWF is also a great example where collaboration is at the heart of work to address OCSA; this includes the development of tools to detect and remove online CSAM, working with international partners across law enforcement, governments, and technology companies to prevent CSAM being shared and recirculated, as well as a hotline where people can report suspected videos and images displaying CSA (IWF, 2025c). Moreover, collaboration is not restricted to large, national or international organisations. For example, IWF, and Cyacomb (a cyber security company), have recently introduced a pilot that enables smaller platforms to utilise cutting edge tools, enabling them to match content uploaded by users against IWF-known lists of CSAM. This not only ensures users are kept safe, but also helps ensure such platforms are compliant with the Online Safety Act 2023 (IWF, 2024a).

So far, the chapter has considered ways in which technology may be used to identify *known* CSAM. However, what about instances of *unknown* CSAM? This is where the use of Artificial Intelligence (AI) and Machine Learning come into play.

Artificial Intelligence and Machine Learning

AI and machine-learning tools are a vital 'cog' in the fight against OCSA. Such tools typically involve the *proactive* detection of child nudity, and previously unknown exploitative child content. This means a high volume of violating content can be removed (often before being seen), as well as locating accounts engaging in potentially inappropriate interactions with children, to remove them and prevent further harm (Meta, 2018).

Thorn, a non-profit technology company that develops software to tackle CSA on a global scale (Thorn, 2025), utilises classification tools to detect unknown CSAM. This includes material that was already available, but which had not yet been identified as CSAM, as well as text-based CSE, demonstrating their value over tools only able to identify pre-existing CSAM (Thorn, 2023). Because the volume of CSAM and messages heavily outweigh the capacity of human moderators, tools are required to be able to review such material. This is where 'classifiers' come into play. Thorn's classifiers use machine-learning approaches to sort data into categories (akin to the approach used by e-mail 'spam' folders), and identify new/unknown CSAM in images or videos, as well as CSE facilitated through text conversations. This has resulted in 1,546,097 files being identified as potential CSAM in 2023, a rise of 384% from 2022 (Thorn, 2023). Microsoft have joined forces with Thorn, as well as All Tech is Human (a non-profit organisation that promotes collaboration and knowledge sharing to help develop the responsible technology field; All Tech is Human, 2024) and other leading organisations in an initiative to prevent the use of AI in facilitating harms against children. This initiative seeks to develop and train generative AI models that can proactively tackle online child safety; release and share such models once they have been trained and evaluated; and maintain and update such models, to respond dynamically to evolving risk (Microsoft, 2024; Thorn, 2024).

Filtering Technologies

In addition to the use of technological advances to prevent the spread of CSAM, filtering approaches are used to prevent access to potential victims. In Autumn 2024, Meta introduced new privacy settings for teenage Instagram users, for those aged 13 (the sign-up age threshold) to 17. This included designating teenage accounts to private by default, only being able to message or tag such accounts by those accounts they follow/are linked to, and having restrictive settings on sensitive content. Users under the age of 16 would require a parent's permission before editing these settings, though teenagers aged 16 and 17 can amend these without parental consent. Parents now also receive greater control over their children's use of the app, as well as monitoring who they are engaging with. These restrictions and teenage accounts have been implemented initially within the UK, US, Canada and Australia, and the European Union in late 2024, and globally from 2025 (Carroll, 2024).

In addition, social media companies have taken steps to restrict who teenagers can connect with. For example, once potentially suspicious adults are identified on Facebook and Instagram, these platforms subsequently inhibit them from connecting with teenage accounts. This may include not recommending young people's accounts to them by removing such profiles from the 'People You May Know' feature; not allowing such users to comment on the posts of young people, nor view comments left by young people on others' posts; and being unable to 'friend' or follow a young person's account, even if they search for their username directly (Meta, 2025).

Similar approaches have been adopted within online gaming. For example, with SIE, on the PlayStation network, users can engage in a number of activities that link them with others; this involves playing games with other users, using text, voice or video chat, sending photos, or joining online communities relating to specific games, or topics (Sony Interactive Entertainment, 2025c). However, parents are able to effectively 'manage' children's accounts, creating separate accounts for each child, adapting their profile to ensure they can only access age-appropriate content, as well as controlling how long they can play games, whether they can share photos or videos with other users, and whether/how much they can spend at the PlayStation online store (Sony Interactive Entertainment, 2025c). Moreover, users that experience inappropriate behaviour can mute players during a game, prevent them from viewing their profile or contacting them, or limit their ability to play with them in future (Sony Interactive Entertainment, 2025d).

Discussion of such filtering technologies has demonstrated how human intervention can capitalise on features embedded within platforms to restrict perpetrators' access to victims. Such approaches are also evident with schemes where users can remove material themselves, i.e. through the 'Take It Down' portal.

Take It Down Portal

The *Take It Down* Portal was developed by the National Center for Missing and Exploited Children, with support from Meta. The portal works by providing users the opportunity to help remove or prevent the online sharing of nude, partially nude, or sexually explicit material of them taken when they were under the age of 18, that they believe have been, or may be, shared online (NCMEC, 2025b). The portal works on either public, or unencrypted platforms that have agreed to take part. The system works by assigning a unique 'hash value', or digital fingerprint, to nude, partially nude, or sexually explicit images or videos of people under the age of 18, which can be used to identify any replica images or videos on the platforms of participating companies, and then to remove such content (NCMEC, 2025b). However, at the time of writing, only twelve platforms have signed up to utilise such technology (NCMEC, 2025c).

The Take it Down portal has been derived based on successes with similar mechanisms, i.e. StopNCII.org, which supports adults to prevent the sharing of intimate images online. StopNCII.org utilises the same technology as the approach used by Take It Down, in assigning a hash value, or unique digital fingerprint, to images, which is then shared with participating companies so they can identify and remove such images from being shared. The Take It Down initiative also shares similarities with the 'Report Remove' tool, which is a UK service for people under 18 to report and remove sexually explicit images or videos of themselves. This is a collaboration between the IWF and Childline (which is provided by the NSPCC) and provides an anonymous method for young people to report explicit material of themselves, for this to be taken down (IWF, 2025d).

Reporting Mechanisms

There exist multiple reporting mechanisms across platforms, where users can report instances of violating content/breaches of a site's code of conduct. As noted earlier, technology is used to proactively detect and remove violating material from platforms, often before being seen by anyone. However, for violating material that *does* make its way onto platforms, human reviewers and technology work in conjunction to review reports submitted by users. Sometimes such reviews will be performed automatically by technology, without human input, with action taken immediately (Meta, 2024a). This has addressed previous issues whereby human reviewers would spend a significant amount of time reviewing content, often on lower-level or even non-violating content, meaning they had less time to spend reviewing more extreme content. This has meant that human reviewers are now able to spend additional time on more nuanced, complex and harmful content, where human reviewers tend to outperform technology.

With YouTube, human reviewers can swiftly remove violations flagged up by their systems or by their users and trusted flaggers, and with Meta, the use of human input is required where technology may miss something, or require further information (Google, 2024; Meta, 2024b). Within an online gaming context, i.e. SIE, human moderation teams support players across all languages on a 24/7 basis, wherever PlayStation Network services are accessible (Sony Interactive Entertainment, 2025e). SIE encourage users to report content in breach of their code of conduct (Sony Interactive Entertainment, 2025b). Upon receipt of a user report, moderation teams carefully review the report and decide on appropriate action. Where a report is upheld, content will be removed and appropriate action taken; this can include written warnings, or suspension of a player's account from the PlayStation Network (Sony Interactive Entertainment, 2025b, d, e). In addition to action being taken on a user's account, reports can also be escalated for further review; for example, to law enforcement authorities (or other appropriate agencies) if the conduct of a user(s) involves the threat to life, the threat to safety of a reporting user or another person, or represents conduct that is believed by SIE to be unlawful (Sony Interactive Entertainment, 2025b). SIE ensure transparency of this process by conveying details of decisions to those involved, and providing a process of appeal in the case of permanent suspension, where appropriate (Sony Interactive Entertainment, 2025e).

It is of note that the technology and models used by technology organisations are enhanced continually over time as they receive further examples of violating content (Meta, 2024a), building their capacity to detect and remove more nuanced and complex material as they receive additional detail on human decisions taken.

As noted above, both technology and human moderation teams can review content reported as violating a platform's community standards. Such content may be reported by users, or by 'trusted flaggers'.

Trusted Flagger Programmes

Trusted, or priority-flagger programmes help provide specific tools to government agencies, or non-governmental organisations, to help them report violating content on platforms. Such groups would typically commit to the regular reporting of violating content on a platform, and tend to exhibit a high degree of effectiveness and accuracy on content reported. Content reported by priority or trusted flaggers is not dealt with differently to content reported by standard users, nor is it automatically removed, though such flagged content is typically prioritised due to the high extent of accuracy (Google, 2025). For further details on guidelines and best practice in UK 'Trusted Flagger' programmes, please refer to the UK Safer Internet Centre (2023).

Use of Global Partners

Social media organisations engage regularly with global partner organisations; for example, Meta's Trusted Partner programme, to support their monitoring efforts and capabilities, drawing on, '…over 400 non-governmental organisations, humanitarian agencies, human rights defenders and researchers from 113 countries around the globe' (Meta, 2023). In addition to global support through the monitoring of content, local partners work with social media organisations to share local knowledge and expertise that help feed into policy, enabling the effective implementation of tailored policies across global (and local) contexts (Meta, 2023).

Challenges in the Fight Against Online Child Sexual Abuse

Though there have been a multitude of advancements in the fight against OCSA, there remain a degree of complex challenges that threaten the successful implementation of such measures; this section will now consider some of these challenges.

End-To-End Encryption

End-to-end encryption has been introduced by some social media companies and messaging platforms to help ensure privacy for users, ensuring only senders and receivers of messages can access message content (Meta, 2024c). However, critics (including the UK Government, and the IWF) argue that if such changes are rolled out more widely without putting necessary child safety measures in place, such platforms will no longer be able to identify, report and stop the spread of CSAM shared within encrypted messages (IWF, 2025e; Gov.uk, 2023a, b).

At the time of writing this chapter, there has been no indication that these social media companies intend to reverse any changes regarding the use of end-to-end encryption. The Virtual Global Taskforce[7] has called on industry partners to fully appreciate the fallout such measures will have, essentially, '…blindfolding themselves to CSA occurring on their platforms', and to take steps to address this issue (Virtual Global Taskforce, 2024).

Age Verification and Filtering Technologies

Age verification is an ever-present issue with regards to users setting up online profiles, and particularly the process of self-verification. In 2019, Instagram began asking new users for their age when signing

[7] The Virtual Global Taskforce is an international alliance of 15 dedicated law enforcement agencies working alongside affiliate members from private industry and non-governmental organisations to tackle the threat of CSA (Virtual Global Taskforce, 2024).

up (Meta, 2022). Historically, age-verification processes have typically involved inputting a date of birth to verify a user is over the permitted age for a platform; a task which, unfortunately, is not difficult to circumvent. This has led to several under-age users subscribing to such platforms, bypassing such verification processes, which essentially become futile. Indeed, it has been reported by Ofcom that over a fifth (22%) of 8–17-year-olds report that they are aged over 18 in order to access social media apps (McMahon et al., 2024).

It is, however, of note that there has been a shift in the use of age-verification approaches. For example, in recent years Instagram have begun to test new age-verification methods. Specifically, if someone attempts to edit their date of birth from under 18 to over 18, they will have three options to verify their age; to provide ID, to ask others to 'vouch' for their age, or to use technology that confirms their age based on a short video of them (Meta, 2022).

However, what about children who say they are over 18 from the start? Such options apply to those attempting to change their date of birth from under 18 to over 18, rather than those who state they are over 18 from the outset. Instagram have highlighted how they are developing systems to address this; for example, using AI to estimate peoples' ages based on items such as 'Happy Birthday' posts. If a user states they are above a particular age, but Instagram systems indicate otherwise, users will be provided a suite of options to verify their age (Meta, 2021). Such verification and methods may come under further scrutiny as the Online Safety Act 2023 is implemented from 2025, and technology platforms are held to account for material hosted on their platforms.

Rise of Generative AI

Generative AI refers to deep-learning models capable of creating new content; that is, high-quality text, images, or other content, based on data they were trained with (IBM, 2023). The rise of generative AI is constantly evolving, and has led to the growing mass distribution/sale of (life-like) CSAM (Singhateh, 2024; Crawford & Smith, 2023). To give some context and detail around the nature of this issue, work by the IWF has found over 3,500 new AI-generated CSA images uploaded to the same dark web forum as analysed previously in October 2023, with more images in the most serious category of CSAM, the emergence of AI-generated CSA videos, and a noticeable increase in AI-generated CSAM imagery on the mainstream web, including of known victims, and famous children (IWF, 2024b). Moreover, though CSA images are illegal, the tools used to generate so-called 'deepfake' CSA images currently remain legal. Offenders take images of actual victims, using these to refine AI models to create new CSAM, which are often realistic enough to be considered under the same laws as real CSAM (Sky News, 2024; IWF, 2024b). The IWF has offered technology companies that develop generative AI models the opportunity to partner with them, to help prevent their AI technology being used to produce CSAM (IWF, 2025f).

Richard Collard, Associate Head for Child Safety Online Policy at the NSPCC, stated, "The speed with which AI-generated child abuse is developing is incredibly concerning but is also preventable. Too many AI products are being developed and rolled out without even the most basic considerations for child safety." (Collard, cited in Sky News, 2024). Consequently, it will be vital for child safety to be a key consideration within future legislation around AI safety.

The Cost of Human Moderation

This chapter has discussed how human moderation is used to support organisations in making complex decisions on more nuanced content, with such decisions being used to further train generative AI models to enhance their decision-making capabilities on future cases. However, such moderation comes at a price. The explosion of CSAM, particularly that which is generated using AI, has become overwhelming for law enforcement, placing increasing demand on technology companies to enhance their moderation capabilities (McQue, 2024). The work carried out by social media companies in reviewing content is not just performed by staff directly employed by such organisations; this is also outsourced to external companies. This has, historically, resulted in legal cases being brought against social media companies for the impact this has had on staff welfare.

Conclusions: Where to Go from Here

This chapter has considered the complex nature of OCSA, and the work of (and challenges faced by) organisations in the fight against OCSA. Such a complex and multi-faceted crime, especially when framed as a global public health issue, requires a similarly complex and co-ordinated response; set out below are areas that will be key in the fight against OCSA.

Collaboration

This chapter has explored how collaboration is a central feature of efforts to tackle OCSA; for example, in the sharing of technology, coming together as part of specific initiatives, or as part of broader partnerships/alliances. What will be vital going forward is that all relevant groups come together and join forces as part of these initiatives; this includes technology companies, governments, and charity organisations, to address this "whole of society issue" (Microsoft, 2020). This also requires input from smaller, localised organisations, that can help provide localised context and insights to a global problem.

Holding Technology Companies to Account

With the implementation of the Online Safety Act 2023, pressure needs to be placed on technology companies to ensure they are fulfilling their duties to take action to prevent and disrupt OCSA from occurring on their platforms, holding them to account for any violating content held on their platform. However, it remains vital that technology organisations are not just 'seen' to comply with regulations, but are taking active steps to address this. Indeed, in light of the recently published figures of online CSAM (IWF, 2025a), and the implementation of the Online

Safety Act 2023, the IWF have written to Sir Keir Starmer, the current Prime Minister, to intervene and ensure that the Online Safety Act 2023 does not enable criminals to exploit loopholes in these regulations (IWF, 2025a). Specifically, IWF Chair Catherine Brown has urged stronger legislation, alongside a more robust interpretation of the rules by Ofcom:

> "We are deeply concerned that the Codes allow services to remove illegal content only when it is 'technically feasible', which will incentivise platforms to avoid finding ways to remove illegal content in order to evade compliance… the Act does not mandate companies to moderate content uploaded in private communications. As a result, illegal content that is blocked elsewhere on the internet can still be freely shared in private online spaces."
> (IWF, 2025a).

Addressing the Rise of Generative AI

The evolution of generative AI has led to a surge in the production of AI-generated CSAM, often realistic enough to be considered under the same legal framework as actual CSAM. Moreover, just as AI is being used to train and build on responses and moderation of CSAM, it is also being used to enhance AI models that create new CSAM. More needs to be done to ensure that AI products that are being developed have clear considerations for child safety embedded within them; for it is imperative that child safety is a central focus within any future legislation brought out around AI safety (Collard, cited in Sky News, 2024).

The Need for a Multi-Faceted Response in the Fight Against Online Child Sexual Abuse

This chapter has focused predominantly on the role that can be played by technology companies in the fight against OCSA. However, technology companies represent only a small subsection of groups required to tackle this crime. Indeed, there are a multitude of groups that can help in this fight, including parents/caregivers, young people and peers, schools, technology companies, internet providers, credit card companies, researchers, courts, child protection services, and NGOs (amongst many others; Smallbone & Wortley, 2017). The nature of this crime as a global public health issue requires a combination of primary, secondary and tertiary activities that target not only offenders, but also victims, and settings, in order to prevent OCSA (Smallbone & Wortley, 2017). OCSA is an endemic global public health issue, and as such requires a global, sustained and multi-faceted response to disrupt and prevent this from happening against young people; indeed, the future of our society.

References

Ali, S., Haykal, H. A., & Youssef, E. (2023). Child sexual abuse and the internet—a systematic review. *Human Arenas, 6*, 404–421. https://doi.org/10.1007/s42087-021-00228-9

All Tech is Human. (2024). *About ATIH* [online]. Available from: https://alltechishuman.org/aboutatih

Carroll, M. (2024). Major Instagram update to give parents more control with new teen privacy settings. *Sky News* [online]. 17 September. Available from: https://news.sky.com/story/teenage-instagram-users-to-get-strict-privacy-settings-automatically-in-major-new-update-13216663

Child Exploitation and Online Protection. (2024). *What is online child sexual abuse and exploitation?* [online]. Available from: https://www.ceop.police.uk/Safety-Centre/what-is-online-child-sexual-abuse/

Childlight. (2024). *Into the light index* [online]. Available from: https://intothelight.childlight.org/

Cohen, L. E., & Felson, M. (1979). Social change and crime rate trends: A routine activity approach. *American Sociological Review, 44*(4), 588–608. https://doi.org/10.2307/2094589

Crawford, A., & Smith, T. (2023). Illegal trade in AI child sex abuse images exposed. *BBC News* [online]. 28 June. Available from: https://www.bbc.co.uk/news/uk-65932372

Data Driven Innovation. (2024). *Childlight publishes groundbreaking global index on child exploitation and abuse prevalence* [online]. 27 May. Available from: https://ddi.ac.uk/childlight-publishes-groundbreaking-global-index-on-child-exploitation-and-abuse-prevalence/

Google. (2024). *Fighting child sexual abuse online* [online]. Available from: https://protectingchildren.google/intl/en_uk/

Google. (2025). *About the YouTube priority flagger programme* [online]. Available from: https://support.google.com/youtube/answer/7554338?hl=en-GB

Gov.uk. (2023a). *UK children and adults to be safer online as world-leading bill becomes law* [online]. 26 October. Available from: https://www.gov.uk/government/news/uk-children-and-adults-to-be-safer-online-as-world-leading-bill-becomes-law

Gov.uk. (2023b). *End-to-end encryption and child safety* [online]. 20 September. Available from: https://www.gov.uk/government/publications/end-to-end-encryption-and-child-safety/end-to-end-encryption-and-child-safety

Gov.uk. (2025a). *Online safety act: Explainer* [online]. 24 April. Available from: https://www.gov.uk/government/publications/online-safety-act-explainer/online-safety-act-explainer

Gov.uk. (2025b). *Draft statement of strategic priorities for online safety* [online]. 8 May. Available from: https://www.gov.uk/government/publications/draft-statement-of-strategic-priorities-for-online-safety/draft-statement-of-strategic-priorities-for-online-safety

IBM. (2023). *What is generative AI?* [online]. 20 April. Available from: https://research.ibm.com/blog/what-is-generative-AI

IWF. (2023). *IWF annual report 2023* [online]. Available from: https://www.iwf.org.uk/annual-report-2023/

IWF. (2024a). *New pilot shows way for smaller platforms to play big part in online safety* [online]. 19 December. Available from: https://www.iwf.org.uk/news-media/blogs/new-pilot-shows-way-for-smaller-platforms-to-play-big-part-in-online-safety/

IWF. (2024b). *Artificial Intelligence (AI) and the production of child sexual abuse imagery* [online]. Available from: https://www.iwf.org.uk/about-us/why-we-exist/our-research/how-ai-is-being-abused-to-create-child-sexual-abuse-imagery/

IWF. (2025a). *Call for Prime Minister to intervene as IWF uncovers record levels of online child sexual abuse imagery* [online]. 22 January. Available from: https://www.iwf.org.uk/news-media/news/call-for-prime-minister-to-intervene-as-iwf-uncovers-record-levels-of-online-child-sexual-abuse-imagery/

IWF. (2025b). *Who we are* [online]. Available from: https://www.iwf.org.uk/about-us/who-we-are/

IWF. (2025c). *About us* [online]. Available from: https://www.iwf.org.uk/about-us/

IWF. (2025d). *Report remove* [online]. Available from: https://www.iwf.org.uk/our-technology/report-remove/

IWF. (2025e). *End-to-end encryption and keeping your child safe online* [online]. Available from: https://www.iwf.org.uk/resources/end-to-end-encryption-and-keeping-your-child-safe-online/

IWF. (2025f). *Protect your generative AI models from the devastating harm caused by online child sexual abuse* [online]. Available from: https://www.iwf.org.uk/membership/benefits-of-membership/generative-ai-model-providers/

Lanier, M. M. (2010). Epidemiological Criminology (EpiCrim): Definition and application. *Journal of Theoretical and Philosophical Criminology, 2*(1), 63–103.

McMahon, L., Singleton, T., & Hayes, G. (2024). 'It's so easy to lie': A fifth of children use fake age on social media. *BBC News* [online]. 28 November. Available from: https://www.bbc.co.uk/news/articles/cn4v52ezx17o

McQue, K. (2024). AI is overpowering efforts to catch child predators, experts warn. *The Guardian* [online]. 18 July. Available from: https://www.theguardian.com/technology/article/2024/jul/18/ai-generated-images-child-predators

Merry, O. J., & Whitfield, K. C. (2024). The landscape of sexual harm in the video game, streaming, and esports community. *Journal of Interpersonal Violence, 40*(13–14), 3307–3332. https://doi.org/10.1177/08862605241271349

Meta. (2018). *Facebook: New Technology to Fight Child Exploitation* [online]. 24 October. Available from: https://about.fb.com/news/2018/10/fighting-child-exploitation/

Meta. (2021). *Asking people for their birthdays* [online]. 30 August. Available from: https://about.instagram.com/blog/announcements/asking-people-for-their-birthdays

Meta. (2022). *Introducing new ways to verify age on Instagram* [online]. 23 June. Available from: https://about.instagram.com/blog/announcements/new-ways-to-verify-age-on-instagram

Meta. (2023). *Bringing local context to our global standards* [online]. 18 January. Available from: https://transparency.meta.com/en-gb/policies/improving/bringing-local-context/

Meta. (2024a). *How Meta prioritises content for review* [online]. 12 November. Available from: https://transparency.meta.com/en-gb/policies/improving/prioritizing-content-review/

Meta. (2024b). *How review teams work* [online]. 12 November. Available from: https://transparency.meta.com/en-gb/enforcement/detecting-violations/how-review-teams-work/

Meta. (2024c). *End-to-end encryption on messenger explained* [online]. 28 March. Available from: https://about.fb.com/news/2024/03/end-to-end-encryption-on-messenger-explained/

Meta. (2025). *Online child protection* [online]. Available from: https://about.meta.com/actions/safety/onlinechildprotection/

Microsoft. (2020). *Fighting child exploitation as an industry* [online]. 12 June. Available from: https://blogs.microsoft.com/on-the-issues/2020/06/12/fighting-child-exploitation-project-protect/

Microsoft. (2024). *Microsoft Joins thorn and all tech is human to enact strong child safety commitments for generative AI* [online]. 23 April. Available from: https://blogs.microsoft.com/on-the-issues/2024/04/23/microsoft-thorn-all-tech-is-human-child-safety-generative-ai/

Microsoft. (2025a). *Digital safety content report* [online]. Available from: https://www.microsoft.com/en-us/corporate-responsibility/digital-safety-content-report

Microsoft. (2025b). *PhotoDNA* [online]. Available from: https://www.microsoft.com/en-us/photodna?oneroute=true

NCMEC. (2025a). *About us* [online]. Available from: https://www.missingkids.org/footer/about

NCMEC. (2025b). *Take it down: Get started* [online]. Available from: https://takeitdown.ncmec.org/

NCMEC. (2025c). *Take it down: Participating online platforms* [online]. Available from: https://takeitdown.ncmec.org/participants/

NSPCC. (2021). *Our strategy 2021–2031* [online]. Available from: https://www.nspcc.org.uk/about-us/performance-plans-strategy/

NSPCC. (2024). *Social media, online communities and safeguarding* [online]. 11 January. Available from: https://learning.nspcc.org.uk/online-safety/social-media-online-communities-safeguarding

Singhateh, M. F. (2024). UN expert alarmed by new emerging exploitative practices of online child sexual abuse. *United Nations Human Rights: Office of the High Commissioner* [online]. 5 February. Available from: https://www.ohchr.org/en/press-releases/2024/02/un-expert-alarmed-new-emerging-exploitative-practices-online-child-sexual

Sky News. (2024). AI being used to generate deepfake child sex abuse images based on real victims, report finds. *Sky News* [online]. 22 July. Available from: https://news.sky.com/story/ai-being-used-to-generate-deepfake-child-sex-abuse-images-based-on-real-victims-report-finds-13182725

Smallbone, S., & Wortley, R. (2017). Preventing child sexual abuse online. In J. Brown (Ed.), *Online risk to children: Impact, protection and prevention*. Wiley. https://doi.org/10.1002/9781118977545.ch8

Sony Interactive Entertainment. (2025a). *PlayStation network* [online]. Available from: https://www.playstation.com/en-gb/playstation-network/

Sony Interactive Entertainment. (2025b). *PlayStation safety* [online]. Available from: https://www.playstation.com/en-gb/support/safety/

Sony Interactive Entertainment. (2025c). *PlayStation safety for parents* [online]. Available from: https://www.playstation.com/en-gb/support/account/psn-safety-parents-guide/

Sony Interactive Entertainment. (2025d). *Online safety, account security, and privacy* [online]. Available from: https://www.playstation.com/en-gb/privacy-security-safety/

Sony Interactive Entertainment. (2025e). *Online safety* [online]. Available from: https://sonyinteractive.com/en/impact/online-safety/

Technology Coalition. (2023). *Announcing lantern: The first child safety cross-platform signal sharing program* [online]. 7 November. Available from: https://www.technologycoalition.org/newsroom/announcing-lantern

Technology Coalition. (2025). *Who we are* [online]. Available from: https://www.technologycoalition.org/about

Thorn. (2023). *Technical Innovation: How Thorn uses technology to transform child protection with a safer internet* [online]. 11 July. Available from: https://www.thorn.org/blog/how-thorns-csam-classifier-uses-artificial-intelligence-to-build-a-safer-internet/

Thorn. (2024). *Thorn and all tech is human forge generative AI principles with AI leaders to enact strong child safety commitments* [online]. 16 July. Available from: https://www.thorn.org/blog/generative-ai-principles/

Thorn. (2025). *About* [online]. Available from: https://www.thorn.org/about/

TikTok. (2025). *Protecting teens online* [online]. Available from: https://www.tiktok.com/transparency/en-us/protecting-teens/

UK Safer Internet Centre (2023). *Trusted flagger guidelines and best practice* [online]. Available from: https://saferinternet.org.uk/resource/trusted-flagger-guidelines-and-best-practice

Virtual Global Taskforce. (2024). *Statement on end-to-end encryption* [online]. 22 April. Available from: https://www.nationalcrimeagency.gov.uk/statement-on-end-to-end-encryption

Weingraber, S., Plath, C., Naegele, L., & Stein, M. (2020). Online victimization—an explorative study of sexual violence and cyber grooming in the context of social media use by young adults in Germany. *Social Work & Society, 18*(3), 1–13.

WeProtect Global Alliance. (2023). *WeProtect global alliance's global threat assessment, 2023* [online]. Available from: https://www.weprotect.org/global-threat-assessment-23/

WeProtect Global Alliance. (2025). *About the alliance* [online]. Available from: https://www.weprotect.org/about-us/

Yoti. (2021). *Digital identity as a force for good* [online]. Available from: https://www.yoti.com/wp-content/uploads/Yoti_Overview-2021.pdf

6

Building an Informed Workforce to Prevent and Respond to Violence Against Women and Girls

Ella Rees and Helen Bovill

Introduction

Violence against women and girls (VAWG) has been identified as a substantial public health and human rights issue (Fenton et al., 2016) and an unacceptable and preventable issue within society (HM Government, 2021, p. 8). This has been categorised as, "an epidemic of offending against women and girls" (HMICFRS, 2021, p. 1), with deeply harmful impacts on survivors and society. VAWG can include crimes of sexual violence, domestic abuse, honour-based violence, revenge porn, stalking and coercion. It is of note that the authors recognise these crimes are not exclusive to women and girls, and that the UK Government strategy frames VAWG within a cis heteronormative lens

E. Rees (✉) · H. Bovill
University of the West of England, Bristol, UK
e-mail: Ella.Rees@uwe.ac.uk

H. Bovill
e-mail: Helen2.Bovill@uwe.ac.uk

K. McCartan et al. (eds.), *Developing and Implementing a Public Health and Criminological Approach to Tackling Sexual Abuse*, Palgrave Studies in Risk, Crime and Society, https://doi.org/10.1007/978-3-031-93634-0_6

that does not address the needs within the Lesbian, Gay, Bisexual, Trans, Queer and/or Questioning, Intersex and Asexual community (Beetham et al., 2021).

As noted, examples of VAWG include domestic abuse and sexual violence. Office for National Statistics (ONS) figures estimate that 2.1 million individuals, aged 16 and over, have experienced domestic abuse in 2023 (ONS, 2023a). Total domestic abuse-related crimes in England and Wales (excluding Devon and Cornwall[1]) were recorded at 889,918 in 2023, with only 51,288 reaching prosecution (ONS, 2023a). ONS also estimated 1.1 million adults to be victims of sexual assault (including attempts) in the year ending March 2022, with approximately 7.9 million having experienced sexual assault (including attempts) since the age of 16, and 1.9 million adults estimated to be victims of rape (ONS, 2023b). The volume of sexual offences recorded by the police in England and Wales was the highest level recorded, with 193,566 recorded cases in the year ending March 2022, an increase of 31% (or 45,731 cases) compared with the previous year (ONS, 2023b).

The trauma of VAWG may impact physical health and have long-lasting consequences on mental and emotional wellbeing; for example, anxiety, sleep deprivation, PTSD, suicidality (Dokkedahl et al., 2022). Experiencing VAWG can also increase the risk of homelessness, impact on maternal parenting and increase child exposure to trauma (Levendosky et al., 2006). Domestic abuse and coercive behaviours should be treated as reflective of a pattern of abuse, that will likely escalate, rather than being viewed as isolated incidents (Monckton-Smith, 2019, 2021).

The Fight Against VAWG

Police officers are positioned as key personnel in the response to, and prevention of, VAWG. High-profile cases of VAWG within the police, such as the murder of Sarah Everard by Wayne Couzens in 2021 and

[1] Following the implementation of a new IT system in November 2022, Devon and Cornwall Police were unable to supply various crime data for the period, October 2022 to September 2023, including crimes flagged as being domestic abuse related (ONS, 2024).

David Carrick who pleaded guilty to 85 serious sexual offences in 2023, heightened public distrust in the police and responses to VAWG. The recent Angiolini Inquiry reviewed both cases and outlined 16 recommendations for improved guidance, training, building trust and improved reporting, vetting and recruitment within the police (Angiolini, 2024). Also of note is the establishment of charities set up to give greater voice to survivors. For example, Everyone's Invited (2024) & Police ME Too (2024) was founded in 2020 to amplify the voices of survivors of rape and sexual assault, and "Police Me Too" has recently been set up to amplify the voices of survivors' abuse by police.

Universities that provide police training programmes are therefore well-positioned to develop an informed workforce to prevent and respond to VAWG. The work discussed in this chapter forms part of a wider project that involved interviews with 11 university students and five university staff across different fields (including police training programmes, or Police Constable Degree Apprenticeships—hereon in referred as the PCDA) to explore how informed students felt regarding VAWG. This chapter will focus upon interviews conducted specifically with five PCDA students regarding their views on this. Specifically, the chapter will consider gaps in awareness, confidence and knowledge to prevent and respond to VAWG for students and consider what can be done to build an informed workforce to prevent and respond to VAWG. The chapter will firstly consider the alignment of this work within the Epidemiological Criminology framework, before considering student readiness to respond to VAWG and exploring in further detail the project undertaken. The chapter will then discuss the findings from the research, alongside recommendations for police education (and policing) going forward.

Alignment with the Epidemiological Criminology Approach

Epidemiological Criminology (EpiCrim) aligns with the growing recognition that offending, in this case VAWG, is a community, developmental and life course issue (McCartan et al., 2015). By considering crimes committed against women and girls from a life-course perspective, behaviour can be viewed as a product of an individual's experiences, mental health, wellbeing, individual differences and personality (McCartan & Kemshall, 2020; McCartan & Kemshall, 2023). Therefore, it is clear that EpiCrim is relevant for the prevention of crime, responses to crime and the management of those who commit violence against women and girls, e.g., prison, probation and social care.

This chapter explores the readiness of PCDA students to respond to and prevent VAWG. This aligns with the EpiCrim paradigm as an example of secondary prevention, through early detection of VAWG by training police professionals on recognition and response. Front line staff such as police officers are often required to be first responders, to take disclosures and provide support, and are key personnel in the prevention of VAWG, misogyny and gender inequality.

Student Readiness to Respond

The assumption of training aligning to the readiness of police to respond effectively to crime is seen across the literature. Evidence suggests that officers engaging with higher education, as part of the PCDA, develop as critical thinkers and build on analytical skills for a better understanding of complex issues (Norman & Williams, 2017; College of Policing, 2020), such as VAWG, though there are divided opinions across policing and academia with the occupational culture needing to be considered within the structure of training and education of higher education programmes (Cox & Kirby, 2018).

A small-scale study by Norman and Williams (2017) found student officers reflecting that knowledge from their degree contributed positively to an understanding of their roles and functions, with a sense of empowerment and individual professionalism. However, students felt unable to utilise knowledge and skills within their workplace (Norman & Williams, 2017); therefore, a reflection on the implementation of learning and recruitment within a top-down approach should be considered.

The College of Policing (2022) explored PCDA students' experiences and attitudes through the new recruits' survey. The latest iteration of the survey found higher satisfaction with the course and a greater value seen in the education they received compared to prior entry routes; for example, in preparing them for the reality of the role and providing confidence with the role (College of Policing, 2022). This chapter will now discuss the project undertaken with PCDA students on their experiences and ability/readiness to respond to incidents of VAWG.

Details of the Project

The wider research project involved a total of 11 interviews with students from across a range of professional courses, though for the purposes of this chapter only the findings from students enrolled on the PCDA course have been included (a total of five students). In terms of demographics, all five participants identified as White British with four male participants and one female participant. The sample was recruited using non-probability convenience sampling, with students recruited through word-of-mouth and recruitment posters advertising the research across the university campus.

The overall aim of the study was to establish how ready PCDA students are to prevent and respond to VAWG within their careers. Specifically, this project explored three key research questions:

1. Do students understand the context of VAWG within the UK?
2. Do students feel prepared to prevent and respond to VAWG in their chosen professions?
3. How do students think their university courses can prepare them to be ambassadors against VAWG?

Interviews were audio-recorded and conducted through a combination of in-person interviews on university campus and online via Microsoft Teams. Ethical application was also sought and obtained by the university's ethics review committee.

Analysis

Thematic analysis (Braun & Clarke, 2006) was used for analysis of the semi-structured interview data. The researchers followed the six-step protocol for analysis, initially familiarising themselves with the data by making hand-written consolidation notes following each interview (stage one). Following this, each interview was transcribed and anonymised. Each interview was then analysed to generate initial codes and potential themes to identify a pattern of meaning across the qualitative dataset (stages two and three). This took place initially with authors reading all transcripts for familiarisation, meeting to compare initial findings, followed by utilising the Lumivero Nvivo 12 programme to review and define individual codes and overall themes across the dataset (stage four, five) followed by write up of findings (stage six).

Findings and Discussion

This chapter reports on three overarching themes identified through the research: Understanding of VAWG; Prevalence of VAWG; and Responses to VAWG.

Understanding of VAWG

PCDA students had varied knowledge and understanding relating to VAWG, with the majority of knowledge on VAWG coming from a combination of learning on-the-job, personal experiences, and exposure such as through media, and with some university teachings through modules focused on vulnerabilities.

Participants often related VAWG to domestic abuse offences; whilst situated within the response units, call outs to domestic abuse disturbances are frequent, as reflected in national statistics (ONS, 2023a). All participants used domestic abuse as the baseline reference when discussing what VAWG means to them, referencing physical abuse and most having an awareness of other forms: *"emotional or physical, mental*

... harm against women and girls is how I understand it" (P5), *"it's violence, whether that be physical or emotional, specifically targeted to women and girls ... I think it's predominately from men ... I think it's so embedded into society"* (P3). Some participants recognised the depth and prevalence of VAWG in differing scenarios and there was some reference to controlling and coercive behaviours from men towards women being a societal issue, aligning with definitions of VAWG (HM Government, 2021; Hester et al., 2021).

The importance of police comprehension of VAWG is needed for thorough responses (Carrillo, 2021), with SafeLives (2015, p. 15) finding that 85% of victims who pursued support from police and agencies, had to do so on average five times in a 12-month period, before receiving effective support. Having an understanding of the complexities of abuse, patterns of escalation and what the appropriate interventions are, for both victims and those who commit abuse, ensures that police support can be meaningful and has a positive impact for those involved. Responding officers should therefore be positioned to help remove barriers for victims to access support.

Participants also drew on their own experiences regarding social media exposure to incidents of VAWG, with embarrassment and frustration expressed:

> It's just unbelievably embarrassing ... it reflects so badly on the police force, policing in Britain in general, and how it only makes our jobs harder ... those are the kind of things we joined to investigate, not perpetrate ... And I think unfortunately, there are going to be bad eggs everywhere. And some people will slip through the cracks, vetting isn't perfect. And we didn't do it ... it was a criminal who did it, he was not at the point in which he decided to perpetrate that crime, he was not acting as a police officer no matter the fact he used his supposed police powers to do so ... . (P1)

Participants also spoke about this in the context of their own experiences as parents and partners and as members of society: *"I wouldn't want my partner to have to deal with that ... or my daughter during any point in her life"* (P5), *"Being a dad to teenage girls as well, makes me very mindful"* (P2), and, *"I do feel quite strongly about it [VAWG]. And my wife sort of helped me a lot on this as well"* (P3). This suggests empathy from participants due to relating VAWG to women in their lives, demonstrating a shift in attitudes with gender norms where there is a relationship, a commonplace response seen in the literature (Borrell-Porta et al., 2019; Hershcovis et al., 2021).

Participants recognised university teaching as providing further knowledge and depth to the issue of VAWG, with knowledge embedded into some modules focused on vulnerabilities. However, VAWG was not conveyed as being taught as a standalone subject. That being said, participants did report a focus on this during their studies, *"...at university, there's definitely an emphasis on treating ... domestic violence and domestic abuse incidents as really, really important"* (P1). All participants had an awareness of safeguarding procedures around domestic abuse (such as protection orders) and onward signposting to local organisations, for appropriate support, *"there's so much of that in terms of safeguarding"* (P1). However, participants consistently stated that the majority of learning and comprehension of the scope of VAWG does not come from university teachings and that there is a disparity between how students are taught to understand and respond to VAWG compared to the reality of how they may be able to respond within the restraints of their roles as responders, also found in Norman and Williams' (2017) study.

Prevalence of VAWG

When discussing VAWG within the police, participants referred to the Metropolitan Police, reporting case studies and examples of "what not to do" that were shared as part of induction and training, as well as within university teaching. Higher education (HE) and training can align officers to respond more effectively, through development of critical thinking and understanding of complex issues (Cox & Kirby, 2018). This said, the application of critical thinking and theories of crime and prevention can be hard to practically embed within the day-to-day role of officers, found in this study and by others (Norman & Williams, 2017). Nonetheless, the preparedness of officers to respond to VAWG is outlined in the HMICFRS (2021) report, stating that strategic buy-in is needed to ensure alignment and communication with relevant strategies, including national and local force responses to VAWG. The College of Policing's (2022) survey on PCDA students' experiences found greater value in education and training provision enabling officers to feel more able to respond to the high prevalence of VAWG within their working roles.

Male participants reported they had no exposure to VAWG within their workplace and emphasised that the workplace is built on a sense of equality and that teams within the force, such as response teams, often feel *"close knit"* and *"like a family"* (P4). Participants noted that boundaries have dropped and there is less *"walking on eggshells"* (P1) with colleagues, *"I think it's gone away from people being so aware of saying the wrong thing, they don't say anything, to being like, we're all friends here, we know where the line is"* (P1).

There were, however, accounts of VAWG that female colleagues have endured by the public, *"I've seen female officers assaulted by members of the public"* (P1). One participant also reflected on how male suspects can have a heightened response to female officers compared to men, a further indication of gender norms and views of male-centric professions, *"one chap got arrested by a female officer … and he flatly refused to go out to the police car unless he was taken out by a male police officer because he thought that was going to be demeaning to his ego"* (P2).

A female participant recalled incidents of VAWG experienced by women within the police, with reference to the murder of PCSO Julia James, *"I think that was the first time I was like, oh, I'm not invincible at work … I don't see VAWG internally as a big issue, but as an outsider, I definitely feel vulnerable in my role that people can target me for being a police officer"* (P3).

One participant also spoke about male-dominated spaces in the police, with operational roles such as firearms, and how there was an internal push for more female colleagues to join such teams, but that female officers did not feel included in these environments, *"I think it is because there is more of an old man sort of club … a lot of female officers that went up there didn't feel too included"* (P3), indicating there are still issues with gender roles within the police. The independent review of the Metropolitan Police identified a culture within this workforce, *"the presence of everyday sexism and misogyny within the Met is well known*" (Casey, 2023, p. 274).

Reiner (2010) explored police culture by highlighting how informal norms, values and attitudes shape policing practices beyond official policies, emphasising how occupational pressures, socialisation and group identity can influence officers' behaviours. One key aspect Reiner discusses is the concept of *canteen culture*, which refers to the informal conversations and shared beliefs amongst police officers, often reinforced in social settings like break rooms or police canteens (Reiner, 2010). Defined as, "*a term frequently used to sum up attitudes (often racist and sexist) that prevail among workers within an organisation, despite these attitudes being officially disapproved of by the organisation they work for*" (HMICFRS, 2023), canteen culture can sometimes foster solidarity and camaraderie, but it can also perpetuate problematic attitudes such as sexism and a resistance to external scrutiny. This may in turn create an environment in which VAWG is able to exist. When discussing canteen culture, participants did not feel this is an issue that they have been exposed to within the workplace, *"I've never heard anything that has been inappropriate, in the way that between friends, it's not inappropriate … I guess you talk to your friends and colleagues in a different way that you would talk to [the] public"* (P1).

Whistleblowing procedures to report inappropriate behaviour by colleagues are outlined within each police force and the Code of Practice for Ethical Policing (College of Policing, 2023, p.4), however, the close-knit makeup of teams is an issue for those potentially reporting colleagues and in establishing boundaries of what is deemed "acceptable" behaviour. This "closeness" may in turn blur the lines of what is deemed acceptable behaviour, including jokes and "banter", with the occupational culture of policing fostering loyalty amongst officers that may discourage reporting (McCartney & Parent, 2015; Taylor et al., 2024). The interviews highlighted the use of banter and jokes as a coping mechanism, *"the canteen culture was pretty, well, there's quite a lot of banter … the police force is full of quite a lot of banter … there's a lot of gallows humour because it's a way to laugh your way through some pretty horrible things"* (P1).

Responses to VAWG

Participants have evidence-based, victim-focused approaches embedded in their learning in both university and as police officers, aligning with frameworks for VAWG (Avon and Somerset Police, 2022, pp. 3–10; College of Policing and NPCC, 2024, p. 11). VAWG as a concept was described as a *"targeted approach to an issue which is getting … more prevalent in terms of priorities"* (P1), suggesting that VAWG is viewed with importance within the day-to-day responses for police. Participants recalled how university teachings have allowed for the development of critical thinking skills around responding to VAWG, and generally as officers, to ensure understanding and consideration around the impact, *"they make it very, very clear that you need to be as objective as possible"* (P1). The HMICFRS (2021) report and College of Policing and NPCC (2024) framework both give examples of best practice through academic research for knowledge building, critical thinking and evidenced-based approaches to increase preparation and improve responses to VAWG. Academic literature has also highlighted the importance and application of evidence-based policing (Ramshaw & Soppitt, 2018; Watkinson-Miley et al., 2022) and feedback from participants in this study has highlighted the value in university teachings in combination with learning "on-the-job".

As has been highlighted earlier in the chapter, police officers are exposed to a range of violence and may need ways of expressing and relaying the effects this may have. Reflective practice is an embedded practice within the university course and may provide PCDA students the tools to reflect on the personal impact their roles may have, which one participant referenced explicitly, "*Our role is so reactive. I've used what I've learnt … more like a personal reflective basis … I thought, how does it affect me?*" (P2). It is argued that being reflective in the role can aid officers to think analytically (Grint & Thornton, 2015) and can aid long-term prevention of crime (Tilley & Laycock, 2014), as well as strengthening responses to VAWG.

Participants also spoke about their knowledge and application of safeguarding and procedures when attending incidents of VAWG, particularly incidents of domestic violence, with expressions of it being hard to ensure all avenues are addressed when responding to crime:

> There's so many, so many things that we have to do in terms of safeguarding … that we have to do, various charities, social services … I don't think that necessarily means that every time we get it completely right. We do so much more than we have to in a criminal justice perspective … we do so much more than our remit suggest that we do … and sometimes that's not enough. But we do our best. (P1).

When discussing if participants felt they can adequately and appropriately respond to VAWG, in relation to on-the-job responses, all participants felt that had adequate skills and knowledge to engage with those who have committed an offence, and victims, *"in general terms, I was prepared and ready … I probably knew enough to know where to get help and how not to, let's say, mess up the situation when I got there"* (P2).

However, participants also expressed that, as previously mentioned, there is a disconnect between teaching someone "how to be a police officer" and responding appropriately to all "jobs", considering the protocols that must be followed and the workload intensity for responding officers, *"I don't really think, at the end of the day, you can train someone for what it is … when you'd experience … those sort of things … there's a level of detachment, almost like a personal detachment … when I'm in the uniform … it almost helps dissociate"* (P3). In such instances, officers may be positioned as responding to a "job" and do not necessarily view themselves as positioned to tackle and dismantle VAWG. This also draws attention to how officers may process and cope with the violence they are exposed to in their roles, with high levels of vicarious trauma, a topic often discussed in the literature (Foley et al., 2022).

This said, one participant said they felt VAWG was a *"political issue"* and that police *"should definitely stay away"* from political issues, positioning themselves as an advocate against VAWG, by being in the role of an officer:

> I don't know if I even have to do much more than what I already do, just by being a police officer … I don't feel like I have to particularly champion it any more than just doing the job (P1).

Participants also spoke about diversity within the police that greater diversity in gender, sexuality, race and cultural understandings, would allow for more appropriate and understanding responses to VAWG:

> I've been to a job where even though my training was about making sure that we get to the bottom of things … a female victim found everything that me and my colleague said offensive … the fact that we weren't a police officer who was a woman of South Asian descent, which meant in her eyes, we were part of the problem (P1).
>
> I do find that some of the older officers … have more traditional views … and some of those traditional views … we wouldn't be very comfortable with… As the PCDAs come into the force, and as the profile gets slightly younger … and as it becomes more diverse, whether that's ethnically or indeed from a gender perspective … I do think that's probably where some of the issues may lie in terms of some of those outdated views (P2).

One participant suggested pairing male and female responding officers to incidents of sexual violence, believing that the combination of male and female approaches with victims "*allows you to deal with a range of situations, you can complement each other*" (P2).

It was also discussed that a lack of diversity and appropriate responses to VAWG has increased public distrust, with participants stating that "*…in my policing, I want to be at least one person who is of a certain age, a certain gender and a certain ethnicity, who can demonstrate that actually, I'm open minded and progressive*" (P3), and, "*…we probably need a more diverse police force. But that's a separate issue*" (P1). A more diverse police workforce in terms of age, gender, sexuality, race, ethnicity, religion, will allow for greater understanding and a more representative response to VAWG, also noted in the government's VAWG strategy (HM Government, 2021, p. 66). Williams and Sondhi (2022) argue that a more diverse police workforce will also allow for reinforcement of the *civic* aspect of policing to understand and communicate effectively across diverse community settings, nurturing the public-health and public-value drive needed in the current climate.

All participants reported that where incidents of VAWG and misogyny may occur within the workplace, they would respond by calling out behaviours and reporting to seniors, where appropriate. This said, the power imbalances within the rank structure of the police, and close-knit makeup of teams, could make responding more difficult:

> I do think there is an issue with groupthink, people wanting to fit in and this is where you've got a challenge here ... You've got small, fairly close-knit teams, where for you career progression, you rely upon the approval of a sergeant and a supervisor, are you going to cause a lot of problems ... you're going to be seen as a bit of a troublemaker ... (P2).
> It's a close-knit little community ... sort of a family ethos ... they do try and deal with things internally quite a lot (P5).

One participant recalled how their female colleagues are "*some of the feistiest*" (P2) they knew, due to high levels of banter, which they stated could be due to the amount of "*misogynistic quips*" (P2) made towards them. This participant then reflected:

> Is that because there is a groupthink, sort of, male dominated thinking in the police, and those women have decided that they will almost play by the rules of that culture? (P2).

This reflection gives insight into a presence of a male-centric space within the police and raises questions around how the police can effectively and appropriately respond to VAWG in their communities, if VAWG-supportive attitudes can be perpetuated within the police force. National College of Policing (2023, p. 5) published insights into VAWG across police forces in the UK, finding 1483 individual reports of police perpetrated VAWG, against 1539 officers, between 1 October 2021 and 31 March 2022, though it's noted the true scale of incidents is believed to be higher. Our participants recalled misogyny, particularly "banter", being present within their workforce. Working towards diminishing any gender stereotypes, by both men and women, and ensuring efficacy in policing, should increase public confidence and increase the effectiveness of support by the police towards victims of VAWG. Theory and critical thinking skills embedded into the PCDA also provides the opportunity to tackle stereotypes and develop critical knowledge around the epidemic prevalence of VAWG in our communities and positions police officers to more effectively respond and tackle VAWG within their roles.

Conclusion and Recommendations

This chapter outlined findings from a small-scale study exploring PCDA students' readiness to prevent, and respond to, VAWG. Developing an informed workforce through university education can help position police to be better equipped to respond to the needs of their communities, including development of critical thinking, reflective practice and prevention-centred, public-health responses to VAWG. The findings are summarised below in the context of the research questions explored:

1. Do students understand the context of VAWG within the UK?

PCDA students indicated a range of knowledge and understanding in relation to VAWG, developed through on-the-job learning, personal experience and exposure to the area, i.e. through the media, or module content. VAWG was typically related to domestic abuse offences, though some recognised the breadth and prevalence of VAWG across other contexts. Though this area was a key focus of their studies, participants identified a disconnection between how PCDA students are taught to understand and respond to VAWG, and the realities of this in practice given the restraints of operational demands.

2. Do students feel prepared to prevent and respond to VAWG in their chosen professions?

All participants felt they had adequate skills and knowledge to respond appropriately to those who have committed an offence with respect to VAWG. With respect to victims, participants described knowledge of where victims could access help, though highlighted the difficulties in ensuring all avenues were fully addressed when attending incidents of VAWG and domestic violence. Though participants reported being able to challenge instances of misogyny in the workplace, this may be made more difficult given the presence of power imbalances across teams, and the close-knit nature of police teams.

3. How do students think their university courses can prepare them to be ambassadors against VAWG?

PCDA students have evidence-based, victim-focused approaches embedded in their learning within university and also within their roles in the police, and VAWG has been flagged as a significant issue in operational policing. University courses have supported the development of critical thinking around responding to VAWG, to enhance understanding around the impact of such crimes, however, there remains a disconnect between teaching someone how to "be" a police officer, responding appropriately to all jobs, and the challenges faced in practice. Moving beyond theoretical knowledge and providing opportunities for active engagement in this area will also further strengthen the role of PCDA students as ambassadors against VAWG.

Ultimately, the PCDA has the potential to create a generation of police officers who are informed, prepared and committed to tackling VAWG. The findings from the study highlighted some key recommendations for police education and practice in this area:

Continued Module or Subject Focus on VAWG to Be Embedded into PCDA Courses

Specific and focused teaching on VAWG, either as standalone modules or thoroughly embedded within existing modules, should be key for PCDA curricula moving forward. Ensuring PCDA students have a thorough understanding of the scope of VAWG and the impacts on victims will support them in being able to readily respond and help prevent the perpetuation of violence. Dismantling any existing stereotypes and educating officers on the signs of abuse and the escalations in behaviour will prepare the workforce to be more responsive through raising standards and improvements in the culture, removing barriers for victims and increasing public confidence in the police. Encouraging students to participate in VAWG-related initiatives, community partnerships and advocacy work will also help reinforce their commitment to cultural and institutional change.

Continued Critical Thinking and Reflective Practice to Be Embedded in PCDA Courses

It is recommended that building critical thinking skills, i.e., around theories of crime and public-health approaches, and reflective practices for officers, should be continually embedded in PCDA courses. Participants reported the benefits of applying critical thinking within their daily roles, however, they also acknowledged the difficulties of balancing this with operational demands. Critical thinking and reflective practice should allow space for officers to reflect on their approaches with the public, whilst also ensuring minimisation of vicarious trauma experienced. Actively addressing features such as unconscious bias and ethical decision-making will empower officers to challenge problematic attitudes both within the force and in the wider community, ensuring officers are more appropriately placed to work with both victims and perpetrators of VAWG.

Ensuring a Diverse Workforce in the Fight Against VAWG

This work highlights the importance of ensuring a diverse workforce in the fight against VAWG. Police forces should strive for improved diversity across policing staff, to ensure more effective responses and awareness of the needs of their communities, including more women in strategic and leadership roles as well as more women in typically "male" roles within the police. This will help address the sense of belonging for women within the police and will position forces to more appropriately address VAWG both internally, and within the wider community. By engaging with communities, third-sector organisations and grassroots projects, police will be embedded into their local communities, to understand the needs, cultural considerations and strengths needed to ensure barriers are broken down to ensure effective, preventative, community-led responses to VAWG.

References

Angiolini, E. (2024). *Angiolini inquiry part 1 report.* Available at: https://iipcv-prod.s3.eu-west-2.amazonaws.com/E02740018_Angiolini-Inquiry.pdf. Accessed March 4, 2023.

Avon and Somerset Police. (2022). *Delivery framework violence against women and girls 2022 / 23.* Available at: https://media.aspolice.net/uploads/production/20230228114350/ASP-VAWG-Delivery-Plan-2022-23.pdf. Accessed January 12, 2024.

Beetham, T., Turley, E., Lazard, L., Thompson, L., & Donnelly, L. C. (2021). An intersectional feminist response to the UK government's violence against women and girls 2021–2024 strategy consultation. *Psychology of Women and Equalities Review, 4*(2), 6. https://doi.org/10.53841/bpspowe.2021.4.2.6

Borrell-Porta, M., Costa-Font, J., & Philipp, J. (2019). The 'mighty girl' effect: Does parenting daughters alter attitudes towards gender norms? *Oxford Economic Papers, 71*(1), 25–46. https://doi.org/10.1093/oep/gpy063

Braun, V., & Clarke, V. (2006). Using thematic analysis in psychology. *Qualitative Research in Psychology, 3*(2), 77–101. https://doi.org/10.1191/1478088706qp063oa

Carrillo, D. (2021). Police culture and gender: An evaluation of police officers' practices and responses to domestic abuse. *Journal of Global Faultlines, 8*(1), 69–80. https://doi.org/10.13169/jglobfaul.8.1.0069

Casey, B. (2023). *An independent review into the standards of behaviour and internal culture of the Metropolitan Police Service: Baroness Casey review.* Available at: https://www.met.police.uk/SysSiteAssets/media/downloads/met/about-us/baroness-casey-review/update-march-2023/baroness-casey-review-march-2023a.pdf. Accessed March 21, 2024.

College of Policing. (2020). *Policing Education Qualifications Framework Initial entry routes Learning to date: development and implementation, 2016 to 2019* [online]. Available at: https://assets.college.police.uk/s3fs-public/2021-02/peqf-learning-to-date.pdf (accessed 2nd July 2025).

College of Policing. (2022). *Evaluation of the Police Constable Degree Apprenticeship (PCDA): First interim report*. Available at: https://assets.production.copweb.aws.college.police.uk/s3fs-public/2022-12/New-recruits-survey-December-2022.pdf. Accessed January 29, 2024.

College of Policing. (2023). *Code of practice for ethical policing*. Available at: https://www.college.police.uk/ethics/code-of-practice. Accessed April 27, 2024.

College of Policing, NPCC. (2024). *Policing violence against women and girls—the national framework for delivery: 2024–2027*. Available at: https://www.npcc.police.uk/SysSiteAssets/media/downloads/our-work/vawg/vawg-framework-for-delivery.pdf. Accessed April 20, 2024.

Cox, C., & Kirby, S. (2018). Can higher education reduce the negative consequences of police occupational culture amongst new recruits? *Policing: An International Journal*, *41*(5), 550–562. https://doi.org/10.1108/PIJPSM-10-2016-0154

Dokkedahl, S. B., Kirubakaran, R., Bech-Hansen, D., Kristensen, T. R., & Elklit, A. (2022). The psychological subtype of intimate partner violence and its effect on mental health: A systematic review with meta-analyses. *Systematic Reviews, 11*(1), 1–16. https://doi.org/10.1186/s13643-022-02025-z

Everyone's Invited. (2024). *Survivor testimonies*. Available at: https://www.everyonesinvited.uk/submissions/read. Accessed February 1, 2024.

Fenton, R. A., Mott, H. L., McCartan, K., & Rumney, P. (2016). *A review of evidence for bystander intervention to prevent sexual and domestic violence in universities*. Public Health England. Available at: https://www2.uwe.ac.uk/faculties/BBS/BUS/law/Law%20docs/dvlitreviewproof0.6.forCLR.pdf. Accessed February 22, 2024.

Foley, J., Hassett, A., & Williams, E. (2022). 'Getting on with the job': A systematised literature review of secondary trauma and post-traumatic stress disorder (PTSD) in policing within the United Kingdom (UK). *The Police Journal, 95*(1), 224–252. https://doi.org/10.1177/0032258X219904

Grint, K., & Thornton, S. (2015). Leadership, management, and command in the Police. In J. Fleming (Ed.), *Police leadership: Rising to the top* (pp. 95–109). Oxford University Press.

Hershcovis, M. S., Vranjes, I., Berdahl, J. L., & Cortina, L. M. (2021). See no evil, hear no evil, speak no evil: Theorizing network silence around sexual harassment. *Journal of Applied Psychology, 106*(12), 1834. https://doi.org/10.1016/S0272-7358(96)00047-5

Hester, M., Walker, S. J., & Williamson, E. (2021). *Gendered experiences of justice and domestic abuse: Evidence for policy and practice*. Available at: https://research-information.bris.ac.uk/ws/portalfiles/portal/282693397/FINAL_Gendered_experiences_WA_UoB_July_2021.pdf. Accessed February 4, 2024.

His Majesty's Inspectorate of Constabulary and Fire and Rescue Services. (2021). *Police response to violence against women and girls: Final inspection report*. Available at: https://assets-hmicfrs.justiceinspectorates.gov.uk/uploads/police-response-to-violence-against-women-and-girls-final-inspection-report.pdf. Accessed February 1, 2024.

His Majesty's Inspectorate of Constabulary and Fire and Rescue Services. (2023). *Glossary – canteen culture*. Available at: https://hmicfrs.justiceinspectorates.gov.uk/glossary/canteen-culture/. Accessed February 1, 2024.

HM Government. (2021). *Tackling violence against women and girls*. Available at: https://assets.publishing.service.gov.uk/media/6194d05bd3bf7f054f43e011/Tackling_Violence_Against_Women_and_Girls_Strategy_-_July_2021.pdf. Accessed February 1, 2024.

Levendosky, A. A., Leahy, K. L., Bogat, G. A., Davidson, W. S., & Von Eye, A. (2006). Domestic violence, maternal parenting, maternal mental health, and infant externalizing behavior. *Journal of Family Psychology, 20*(4), 544–552. https://doi.org/10.1037/0893-3200.20.4.544

McCartan, K., & Kemshall, H. (2020). The potential role of recovery capital in stopping sexual offending: Lessons from circles of support and accountability to enrich practice. *Irish Probation Journal, 17*, 87–106.

McCartan, K., & Kemshall, H. (2023). Incorporating quaternary prevention: Understanding the full scope of public health practices in sexual abuse prevention. *International Journal of Offender Therapy and Comparative Criminology, 67*(2–3), 224–246. https://doi.org/10.1177/0306624x211049204

McCartan, K., Kemshall, H., & Tabachnick, J. (2015). The construction of community understandings of sexual violence: Rethinking public, practitioner and policy discourses. *Journal of Sexual Aggression, 21*(1), 100–116. https://doi.org/10.1080/13552600.2014.945976

McCartney, S., & Parent, R. (2015). Ethics in law enforcement [online]. *BCcampus*, 131–132. Accessed March 12, 2024.

Monckton Smith, J. (2019). Intimate partner femicide: Using Foucauldian analysis to track an eight-stage progression to homicide. *Violence Against Women, 26*(11), 1267–1285. https://doi.org/10.1177/1077801219863876

Monckton-Smith, J. (2021). *In control: Dangerous relationships and how they end in murder* (pp.19–163) [online]. Bloomsbury Publishing. Accessed January 14, 2024.

National College of Policing. (2023). *Tackling violence against women and girls—policing performance and insights publication* [online]. Available at: https://www.npcc.police.uk/SysSiteAssets/media/downloads/our-work/vawg/tackling-vawgpolicing-insights-report---policing-insights-report.pdf. Accessed May 4, 2024.

Norman, J., & Williams, E. (2017). Putting learning into practice: Self-reflections from cops. In *European police science and research bulletin: Special conference edition* (pp. 197–203).

NPCC. (2024). *Policing violence against women and girls – the national framework for delivery: 2024 – 2027*. Available at: https://www.npcc.police.uk/SysSiteAssets/media/downloads/our-work/vawg/vawg-framework-for-delivery.pdf. Accessed March 1, 2024.

Office for National Statistics. (2023a). *Domestic abuse in England and Wales overview: November 2023.* Available at: https://www.ons.gov.uk/peoplepopulationandcommunity/crimeandjustice/bulletins/domesticabuseinenglandandwalesoverview/november2023. Accessed February 6, 2024.

Office for National Statistics. (2023b). *Sexual offences in England and Wales overview: Year ending March 2022.* Available at: https://www.ons.gov.uk/peoplepopulationandcommunity/crimeandjustice/bulletins/sexualoffencesinenglandandwalesoverview/march2022. Accessed February 6, 2024.

Office for National Statistics. (2024). *Crime in England and Wales: Year ending September 2023.* Available at: https://www.ons.gov.uk/peoplepopulationandcommunity/crimeandjustice/bulletins/crimeinenglandandwales/yearendingseptember2023#strengths-and-limitations. Accessed November 25, 2024.

Police Me Too. (2024). *Our stories.* Available at: https://police-me-too.co.uk/. Accessed February 1, 2024.

Ramshaw, P., & Soppitt, S. (2018). Educating the recruited and recruiting the educated: Can the new police education qualifications framework in England and Wales succeed where others have faltered. *International Journal of Police Science and Management, 20*(4), 243–250. https://doi.org/10.1177/1461355718814850

Reiner, R. (2010). *The politics of the police* (4th ed.). Oxford University Press.

SafeLives. (2015). *Getting it right first time*. Available at: https://safelives.org.uk/sites/default/files/resources/Getting%20it%20right%20first%20time%20-%20complete%20report.pdf. Accessed April 24, 2024.

Taylor, O. E. V., Philpot, R., Fitton, O., Walkington, Z., & Levine, M. (2024). Police whistleblowing: A systematic review of the likelihood (and the barriers and facilitators) of the willingness of police officers to report the misconduct of fellow officers. *Journal of Criminal Justice, 91*, Article 102170.

Tilley, N., & Laycock, G. (2014). The police as professional problem solvers. In *The future of policing* (pp. 369–382) [Online]. Routledge. Accessed April 14, 2024.

Watkinson-Miley, C., Cox, C., & Deshpande, M. (2022). A new generation of police officers: Experiences of student officers undertaking the police constable degree apprenticeship in one UK police force. *Policing: A Journal of Policy and Practice, 16*(1), 122–134. https://doi.org/10.1093/police/paab062

Williams, E., & Sondhi, A. (2022). A narrative review of the literature on the recruitment of younger police officers in age and in service: What are the implications for the police in England and Wales? *Policing: A Journal of Policy and Practice, 16*(4), 648–662. https://doi.org/10.1093/police/paac001

7

Disclosure of Sexual Violence/Abuse in an Ecological Frame

Jane Meyrick

> It was fear that stopped me.... fear and I think, a deep kind of shock. I didn't want this to have happened to me. I didn't want to believe it had ...I told K I hadn't been raped. I moved into the bottom of a well and I stayed there a long time. First Person Account, (Higson-Sweeney & Meyrick, 2022)

The barriers to disclosure of sexual abuse, sexual violence, child sexual abuse and rape are complex and multifaceted. Factors range across the lives of survivors as individuals, families and communities but also as people within societies, shaped by cultural norms and structural determinants. To understand why any one victim remains silent we have to look across these levels of experience, using a socio-ecological model of cause and effect. Wider determinants of behaviour at individual (micro), community (meso) and societal (macro) levels, first conceptualised by

J. Meyrick (✉)
University of the West of England, Bristol, UK
e-mail: jane.meyrick@uwe.ac.uk

K. McCartan et al. (eds.), *Developing and Implementing a Public Health and Criminological Approach to Tackling Sexual Abuse*, Palgrave Studies in Risk, Crime and Society, https://doi.org/10.1007/978-3-031-93634-0_7

Bronfenbrenner's ecological system (Bronfenbrenner, 1979) inform the framing of sexual violence within an Epi-Crim approach (Lanier, 2010). The first step is to understand the data, how much does it happen, where and to whom. Prevalence allows us to view patterns and what they mean.

Sexual Violence Is Common

Sexual violence and abuse (SV/A) are common experiences, for the year ending March 2020, the Crime Survey for England and Wales estimated 618,000 (2.9%) of women and 155,000 (0.7%) of men aged 16–74 had experienced sexual assault (Office for National Statistics, 2021a, 2021b). Around half of rape victims had been a victim more than once (Office for National Statistics, 2021c), with the number of reported offences almost tripling in recent years (Office for National Statistics, 2021a).

Low Reporting

Whilst SV/A rates are increasing, reporting continues to remain low with an estimated 84% of female survivors not reporting their abuse to the police (Office for National Statistics, 2021c). Research tells us that lower-level sexual harassment or 'non-contact' abuse is generally normalised, expected and just part of being a woman (APPG, 2021). This is not surprising when data shows that of women aged between 18 and 24, 97% have experienced some form of sexual harassment and almost all did not report (APPG, 2021).

> It does happen a lot, but people don't think much of it anymore. It's just like, 'Oh that's happened again'. People just kind of accept it. (Mullany & Trickett, 2018)

Sexual harassment in the criminal justice system is presented as an 'incident', rather than a culminating pattern of behaviour experienced across the landscapes and lives of women and girls (Meyrick et al., 2024b). Data confirms that harassment not only begins at a young age but remains ongoing (APPG, 2021). A pattern that essentially becomes like a lifelong training in normalisation and silencing, one that helps us understand low reporting levels.

Resulting Justice Gap

Low reporting of SV/A creates what has been called a 'justice gap' (Hester & Lilley, 2017). Data for one region, presented below for female only rape show, if the female population (aged 16–74) of Avon and Somerset is approximately 630,111 (Office for National Statistics, 2024), and the equivalent of 0.4% of women aged 16–74 had experienced rape[1] (Office for National Statistics, 2021b), a maximum of 1.55%[2] of estimated cases result in a conviction (39 convictions out of an estimated 2520 cases). Figure 7.1 illustrates the numbers involved within the Avon and Somerset region, across the different stages of such cases within the criminal justice system.

*CSEW female prevalence rate for rape (excluding attempts) aged 16 to 74 is 0.4% (Office for National Statistics, 2021b).

†0.4% of 630,111 female population aged 16–74 mid-2020 Avon and Somerset (Office for National Statistics, 2024) is 2520.

††Rape Monitoring Group force summaries 2019/20 Avon and Somerset Police (HMICFRS, 2021).

‡Cases not separated by gender.

Therefore, current data, particularly criminal justice related statistics, are missing most of the picture. An increasing epidemic of gender-based violence becomes invisible.

---

1 CSEW female prevalence rate for rape (excluding attempts) aged 16 to 74 (Office for National Statistics, 2021b).

2 1.55% is presented as the maximum figure here as the conviction figure of 39 is not disaggregated by gender.

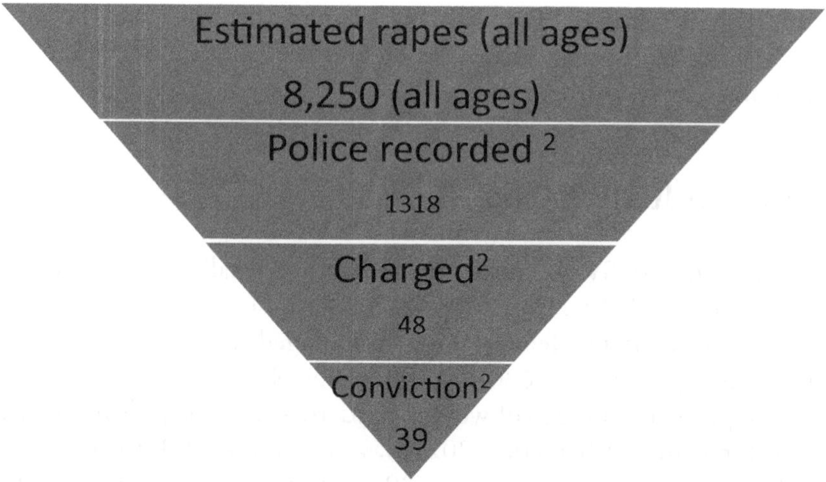

Fig. 7.1 The justice gap: unmet need for rape victims 16+ year up to March 2020
[1] ONS general rate 0.5% (Stripe 2021) by Avon and Somerset Census 1.65 million population, https://www.justiceinspectorates.gov.uk/hmicfrs/police-forces/avon-and-somerset/more-about-this-area/ (HMICFRS, 2023)
[2] Rape monitoring Rape Monitoring Group force summaries 2019/20 Avon and Somerset Police

Trajectory of Harm Impact on Victims—Trauma

The harmful effects of SV/A compounded through silencing and delayed disclosure ripple across generations, affecting individuals' capacity to work, participate in family and community life (Lanthier et al., 2018). Those who have experienced SV/A report poorer health and more use of medical services (Du Mont & White, 2007). Healthcare needs include physical health consequences such as injuries, pregnancy, gynaecological complications (infection, vaginal bleeding, chronic pelvic pain, reproductive issues) (McCormack et al., 2022) and risks of sexually transmitted diseases as well as gastrointestinal injuries (Lanthier et al., 2018).

The routes unprocessed trauma takes through the lives of survivors can be expressed in ongoing coping behaviours such as addiction, self-harm, eating disorders and risky sexual behaviour (Stensvehagen et al., 2023). Furthermore, issues such as insomnia (Rivara et al., 2019) and high levels of PTSD can result in devastating long-term health issues such as heart disease (Jakubowski et al., 2021) and even in premature death (Wang et al., 2023). These harms are amplified through evidence of survivors significant avoidance of healthcare (Hooper & Meyrick, 2025).

In England alone, the cost of all acts of SV/A is estimated to be over 10 billion pounds a year, specifically, for the 120,000 rape offences in 2015/2016, the Home Office estimates the total socio-economical cost (including defensive expenditure, physical and emotional harm, lost output, health and victim service costs and police costs) to be approximately £4.8 billion (Heeks et al., 2018). Money spent is a cold way of capturing harm but crudely reminds us why prevention is so important, particularly for those who do not disclose. Their silence costing a potentially avoidable escalation of unmet need (Combes et al., 2019).

Research evidences the harm of not telling with comparatively more depression and PTSD amongst survivors (Ahrens et al., 2010). Healthcare and support offered to survivors can reduce these long-term consequences but require survivors disclose (Lomax & Meyrick, 2020; O'Doherty et al., 2023). Disclosure can reveal a more accurate picture of SV/A in our society but more importantly, reduce future harm and suffering (Sigurdardottir & Halldorsdottir, 2021). We need to understand telling and what gets in the way.

What Makes It Hard to Tell

Barriers to reporting SV/A span all levels of the ecological or Epi-Crim map of determinants. Reviews of the literature at each level of the ecological system show us how to unpack the complexity of help-seeking (Zinzow & Thompson, 2011).

Fear and Shame

Common feelings of shame and fear of being blamed (Ullman et al., 2010) are effective silencers. SV/A often occurs under circumstances that survivors themselves struggle to describe, such as being spiked, alcohol use (Recalde-Esnoz et al., 2024) or where consent was coerced (Pugh & Becker, 2018). Survivors may struggle to remember details of the assault or fit them into 'acceptable' rape-myth-dominated narratives of rape, making reporting harder (de Souza Costa et al., 2020).

Coerced sex tends to happen with someone you know (Office for National Statistics, 2021c) and lived experience research with survivors in this context show feelings of betrayal, anger, shock and confusion (Higson-Sweeney & Meyrick, 2022). Feelings are often initially directed inwards as survivors blame themselves. Societal 'rape myths' further play into survivors guilt until reporting becomes unthinkable (Peter-Hagene & Ullman, 2018).

> I'm like how the hell can someone do that? Especially like he cared about me, I cared about him…it's insane how someone can inflict that amount of pain and harm. Imogen (Higson-Sweeney & Meyrick, 2022)

Even if the traumatic impact of assault is very deeply felt by the victim, up to 60% of women (Wilson & Miller, 2016) and perhaps even more men (Reed et al., 2020) struggle to acknowledge a rape.

Reactions to Telling

Anticipated negative reactions to disclosure are well founded as research on reactions from family and friends, often reflect victim blaming rape myths (Ahrens et al., 2007). Responses such as 'were you drinking' seek to focus on the contribution of victims' choices.

The anxiety and discomfort of the responder can block disclosure. Research on disclosure of child sexual abuse shows listeners may react by signalling the survivor to stop (McElvaney, 2019).

Informal first steps to telling often produce unhelpful responses, 'You blame me therefore I blame me' (Bonnan-White et al., 2018) and silence future attempts to disclose (Orchowski & Gidycz, 2012). In contrast, positive reactions to disclosure can aid recovery and encourage help-seeking (Ullman & Peter-Hagene, 2014).

Making sense of experiences of sexual abuse and violence is already difficult but our own coping mechanisms may work against us.

Trauma Responses

Sexual violence can set off a 'prolonged crisis', disrupting health and mental health (Van der Kolk, 1994). Survivors' capacity to recognise and articulate their experiences coherently or consistently is undermined by how we cognitively process and recall trauma, often resulting in fragmented recollections or even memory suppression. In turn, such inconsistency is framed as lying by reporting agencies (Herlihy & Turner, 2015).

Survivors are rendered unconvincing and common understandings of what rape and sexual assault looks like, where it happens and how survivors should behave (rape myths) form structural barriers to disclosure. Joining the dots, we need to see this ongoing pattern of not listening or believing for what it is, intersectional social inequality.

Refusing to Hear: Culture and Society

Rape myths underpin how friends and family react to disclosure but also how services, organisations such as health professionals, the police and courts respond to disclosures. Rape myths are the lens through which survivors make sense of their experiences but they also shape agencies decisions about how to handle reporting (Hudspith et al., 2023).

Structural resistance to hearing can be seen in the gulf in language between how survivors describe their experience against professionals' terminology a survivors "problem with consent" vs a agency's 'rape'. The dearth of common victim-centred descriptors show a gap in understanding that actively blocks telling (Ahrens et al., 2010). More importantly, struggling to name it is not just a lack of language but illustrates the hearing-resistant maps we use to understand (Meyrick, 2022).

Society actively reduces SV/A survivors' ability to conceptualise or report their own victimisation.

Vanishing Tricks with Language

The experience of sexual violence is often conflated with the overlapping but separate issue of domestic or intimate partner violence (DV or IPV), carried out in the context of a relationship. Around half of those who experience rape or assault by penetration are victimised by an acquaintance, stranger or family member (Office for National Statistics, 2021c). Conflation of the two effectively wipes out half of all victims through a simple act of not seeing. The implications of language and its power to 'disappear' victimisation is evidenced in action, healthcare services commonly screen for IPV or DV but much less for SV/A (Miller et al., 2021). Asking directly and improving recording is at the heart of better prevention (Campbell, 2008).

Furthermore, systems of visibility such as media reporting and criminal justice, often use language that removes SV/A and DV perpetrators; Louise Casey's devastating review of the Metropolitan Police Force (Baroness Casey of Blackstock, 2023) documents passive wording and removal of 'male violence' in naming the cause of sexual violence. Suppression of disclosure in policing mirrors a whole society's approach to SV/A. Refusing to hear is expressed through the operation of the components of society, namely our organisations and institutions.

Refusing to Hear—Organisational Barriers

Schools, workplaces, universities, police and religious bodies reflect the norms and beliefs of the societies we live in. The way they respond to sexual harassment/abuse directly impact disclosure. Structural barriers to disclosure are greater in male-dominated, hierarchical organisations in which evidence shows sexual harassment/violence may be expected or tolerated for example: the police (Baroness Casey of Blackstock, 2023), healthcare (Cox et al., 2023), higher education (Towl & Walker, 2019), science, technology, engineering and medicine (Committee on the Impacts of Sexual Harassment in Academia, 2018) and the military (Buchanan et al., 2014). Organisational barriers to disclosure include institutional concerns about reputation, an HR focus on minimising consequences for organisations and discouraging complainants, or simply a lack of trust in poor reporting systems. Critically, the pattern of barriers is not uniform but describe intersectional inequality. We know that racially minoritised communities (Burton & Guidry, 2021), people with disabilities (Basile et al., 2016) and members of the LGBTQIA + community (Tillewein et al., 2023) are more likely to be sexually harassed or abused and yet are less likely to tell.

Social inequality ensures that some groups are refused credibility (Armstrong et al., 2018) and that intersections of identity form a 'matrix of domination' (Collins, 2017). Societal racism scaffolds stereotypes that perpetuate disbelief of victims from racially minoritised communities, such as hyper-sexualisation of black women's bodies (Fritz et al., 2021). Marginalised communities mistrust reporting institutions based on direct experience of racism which blocks formal help-seeking (Slatton & Richard, 2020). True inequality lies in the power to render social injustice unobtainable.

Survivors are well aware of the dismissive attitude of society and institutions, research describes a cost–benefit analysis approach to disclosure with questions of 'Will I be believed' and 'Was it my fault' set against clear societal messages, you will not be believed and it was your fault (Schwarz et al., 2017). It is not surprising then that even the United Nations conclude that <u>not</u> reporting is a rational choice (Sen et al., 2018).

How then can survivors hope to be able to report their experience in a way that systems will hear?

Understanding Disclosure as a Process

The evidence around what supports disclosure suffers from a type of scholarly fracture along lines of psychology vs criminology, victim vs perpetrator and child vs adult sexual abuse and violence. Telling is also often presented as an incident, rather than part of an ongoing experience. There are obviously some factors unique to childhood, adolescence and adulthood but synthesis across child sexual abuse (CSA) studies (Brennan & McElvaney, 2020) emphasise the need for victims to become aware or grasp what has happened to them and that this is part of an ongoing process. As with adults, naming it requires a basic education around consent and healthy relationships to recognise when something is wrong, equipping survivors with both the words they need to tell but also the understanding of what they experienced. Historically, sex education mirrored society's beliefs about what is or isn't abuse, who can or cannot be abused and how they should react. For example, gender stereotypes in rape myths create structural barriers that prevent male survivors naming their trauma such as 'men cannot be raped' (Walfield, 2021). Once victimisation is recognised, survivors can move through the process to telling.

Reasons to tell can come from within as the emotional burden or 'pressure cooker' effect overwhelms survivors' ability to remain silent, 'I just came out with it' (McElvaney et al., 2012). Trained professionals can help by 'noticing' signs of distress. Disclosure might also be triggered by a need for justice or the compulsion to protect others; in other words, belief in some benefit. Formal disclosure can be prompted by critical personal transitions (Alaggia et al., 2019), high-profile cases (Amber et al., 2019) or wider social movements such as #MeToo (Alaggia & Wang, 2020).

Prompts to tell can also be as simple as just being asked (McElvaney, 2019). However, it is surprising how much this does not happen, even within systems tasked with safeguarding. Making it safe to tell may come from signals the survivor will be believed. Professional difficulty hearing is often communicated and may stem from realistic concerns of not being able to manage the disclosure or do something about it (Hudspeth et al., 2022). Systems, organisations and the way they enable staff to handle disclosure through training, referral mechanisms and response policies is an important place to begin improving disclosure rates through organisations. Being asked can be crucial, in CSA studies, wanting to be asked was the main reason some survivors attended services (Cossar et al., 2019). Being asked represents permission to tell (Lemaigre et al.,

2017). However, asking in the wrong way can still silence. Common safeguarding practice may block disclosure, for example screening questions such as 'Are you scared of your partner?' limits disclosure to DV only (Meyrick et al., 2024a). Survivors coerced to consent who or felt they could not say no will struggle with questions like 'Did you consent?' Professionals may fear asking will cause harm but in evidence around survivors' experiences of research, they generally reported benefiting from telling their story (Jaffe et al., 2015). Reporting may be the start of recovery and survivors describe active engagement or contributing to prevention as restorative, it gives back what has been taken: voice, control and power (Ungar et al., 2009).

Knowing that disclosure is a process (sometimes lifelong) and not an event, can take the pressure off professionals expecting inquiry leading directly to disclosure. The role of professionals in 'asking' is to supply the knowledge and reassurance that there is somewhere safe to tell when ready, providing the first of a series of stepping-stones. Knowledge that there is somewhere safe, as signalled by well-handled asking, gives survivors control and options. However, if we are to truly reveal the scale of SV/A, we have to move beyond the individual barriers to address the structural.

Wider Determinants of Social/Gender Inequality and Prevention

The terms we use to describe gender-based violence are fragmented such as Violence Against Women and Girls, DV and IPV. However, the evidence base is clear in framing sexual violence and harassment as a wider intersectional gender and social inequality issue. Therefore, the terms and maps we use must encompass a recognition of the purpose of gender-based violence in delivering marginalisation and the hoarding of power.

Societies that promote rigidly defined gender roles or hypermasculinity demonstrate higher rates of gender-based violence (Heilman & Barker, 2018). Mechanisms to supress disclosure can therefore be better understood as policing of gender inequality (Meyrick, 2022). Recognition of the function of sexual violence as a tool of inequality demands we use an intersectional lens and acknowledge that survivors' reporting ability or credibility is suppressed by those same intersectional inequalities.

Research into cultural norms in different communities amplify how unwritten rules silence disclosure of wrongdoing (Alaggia et al., 2019). Work in the US describes how African American women have to navigate a fine line between silence and community loyalty when considering disclosing. Research by McGuffey (2013) found 'strong Black women' stereotypes imposed on survivors who are expected to protect African American male perpetrators (Richie, 2012).

If silencing survivors is part of the mechanisms of retaining power then addressing power imbalance at societal level must be part of the solution. That means working towards authentic diversity not often captured in Equality, Diversity and Inclusion (EDI) performative measures (Meyrick, 2022).

Starting work at the point of reporting sexual violence, or action after the event, is characteristic of the criminal justice approach and misses the opportunity to stop it happening in the first place (primary prevention). Addressing structural determinants of sexual violence and silence requires an ecological model-informed understanding of the disclosure processes and behavioural drivers. Reporting after the fact is the first step in fully recognising the scope and scale of gender-based violence before an evidence base and data-led prevention approach can be realised.

Collecting data and examining patterns is a primary tool of public health prevention and/or the Epi-Crim model. Therefore, asking directly, improving disclosure and recording are at the heart of better prevention.

Earning Disclosure—Compassionate and Effective Listening

The main means of reporting SV/A is often seen as the criminal justice system/police. The UK government's own rape review concluded that survivors using the criminal justice system were being failed (HM

Government, 2021). Protecting civil rights and rebalancing gender inequality, through an effective, victim-centred, criminal justice response (McGlynn, 2022) means compassionate formal reporting. Ground breaking reformation of criminal justice reporting through initiatives such as Operation Soteria (Hohl & Stanko, 2024) has begun removing the traditional focus on the victim's credibility and shifting responses to disclosure onto the perpetrator to scrutinise guilt.

Wider places and spaces in which to disclose include the organisations within which sexual harassment/abuse is often experienced and maintained; organisations that deliver gender equality need to build compassionate listening both for those working in them or those reporting to them. Women report that the landscape of harassment and abuse encompasses where they live, work, study, travel and report (Meyrick et al., 2024b) through an escalating scale of harassment to assault. There is a gap around where to disclose with few compassionate or anonymous options. At the same time, what is seen as reportable, should include the full range of harassment such as non-contact abuse or street harassment (Home Affairs Committee, 2024). Online spaces and image-based abuse have evolved beyond existing legal frameworks and the need to protect against virtual harms has not kept pace (EVAW alliance, 2022).

Disclosure may be driven by the desire to stop the behaviour, protect others and a need to see real consequences for perpetrators and yet available systems are built to not listen. One improvement could be increasing compassionate listening to survivors across the full range of organisational structures.

Earning Disclosure—Organisational Approach

A universal setting in which individual, community and structural barriers to disclosure coalesce are organisations. The diagram (see Fig. 7.2) encompasses a whole organisational approach to preventing gender-based violence and improving reporting. It is derived from both the evidence of what works across an ecological or Epi-Crim approach and the voice of survivors themselves.

Environment	• Community consultation around shared approaches - (with not too) • Prevention training – evaluated vs key outcomes • Review policy/procedures vs key aims - balance (complainant + accused) transparency, timeliness. • Range of reporting mechanisms, compare rates to anonymous prevalence • Model it - diversity at all levels
People	• Tiered, effective, training (taking disclosure, bystander, consent) using a gender transformative frame that amplifies benefits, e.g. social justice, intersection inequality and expect and hold backlash. • Signal openness to disclosure in person centred/culturally sensitive language, symbols. • Case finding – ability to recognise cues and ask (case finding) including scrutiny of anonymous prevalence data for patterns/hotspots. • Systems that can scale up anonymous initial reporting to formal reporting and makes links across incidents/perpetrators.
Responding	• Consistency parallel staff + users' policies. • Diversity in trained responders • Inclusive culturally competent language. • Trauma informed and survivor focused, expert supported. • Set out and deliver on benefits of reporting - visible consequences, complainant protection.
Survivors @Meyrick 2020	• Listen • Believe • UNBLAME • Clear benefits to disclosure evidenced • Restore choice and control - next steps.

Fig. 7.2 Earning disclosure: a whole organisation approach (Meyrick, 2022)

Imagine holding a piece of paper in your hand on which is written your most guarded secret. If you were to hand it to a stranger, what would you fear most? Would you be worried about their intrusive questions, being ignored or that they may tell someone else? What would you look for in that stranger, signs of kindness, compassion? Does it seem they have the power to help you or do they just seem open to listening?

Much of what is described in Fig. 7.2 captures well-researched barriers such as shame and blame. What is new is addressing them in one setting with an emphasis on repeatedly defusing feelings of self-blame or active 'unblaming' within a framework that also tackles the expression of structural inequality through systems and policies.

Conclusions

Research tends to break up disclosure of gender-based violence into incidents and factors but this undermines our understanding of disclosure as a process, built on layers of determinants at individual, social, community and society/cultural levels. Ecological models using these scales of complexity have been developed to describe gender-based violence

(Hagemann-White et al., 2010) and yet real world interventions still tend to cluster around individual determinants. Our understanding and efforts to prevent as well as improve reporting cannot be done without seeing the issue as one of power and inequality in which one persons' experience of sexual violence is not simply an 'isolated incident' (Meltzer, 2023) but the result of structural power played out in survivors' lives. Prevention must therefore work across the same landscapes. The focus on organisations presented here is one way to intervene at a meeting point of determinants, where we work.

Our efforts must focus on the silent who have not been able to tell (Brennan & McElvaney, 2020). We need to recognise survivors' resilience as an asset (Lorimer et al., 2023) and disclosure as a restoration of individual power through voice and agency. Great use of co-produce interventions with survivors is both rewarding and restorative in giving back things that have been taken (Meyrick et al., 2023).

> You feel so degraded and worthless, so to actually feel like you are worthy as a person and as a human being is a real big achievement. (Meyrick & Anning, 2021)

Finally, siloed working at one level of the ecological or Epi-Crim model is not enough without parallel interventions on the structural drivers of intersectional gender inequality, complexity is nothing to fear. Child sexual abuse is well understood as something many survivors don't tell but show. Professional guidance such as 'Spotting the Signs' (Spotting the Signs, 2023) puts the responsibility on the professional to be curious and pick up cues, this basic premise should be extended to all sexual abuse and violence. In summary everyone across the society and communities has a role in the prevention and disclosure of sexual abuse and violence.

References

Ahrens, C. E., Campbell, R., Ternier-Thames, K. M., Wasco, S., & Sefl, T. (2007). Deciding whom to tell: Expectations and outcomes of rape survivors' first disclosures. *Psychology of Women Quarterly, 31*(1), 38–49.

Ahrens, C. E., Stansell, J., & Jennings, A. (2010). To tell or not to tell: The impact of disclosure on sexual assault survivors' recovery. *Violence and Victims, 25*(5), 631–648. https://doi.org/10.1891/0886-6708.25.5.631.

Alaggia, R., & Wang, S. (2020). "I never told anyone until the #metoo movement": What can we learn from sexual abuse and sexual assault disclosures made through social media? *Child Abuse & Neglect, 103*, 104312. https://doi.org/10.1016/j.chiabu.2019.104312.

Alaggia, R., Collin-Vézina, D., & Lateef, R. (2019). Facilitators and barriers to child sexual abuse (CSA) disclosures: A research update (2000–2016). *Trauma, Violence, & Abuse, 20*(2), 260–283. https://doi.org/10.1177/1524838017697312.

Amber, B., Dinh, T. K., Lewis, A. N., Trujillo, L. D., & Stockdale, M. S. (2019). High-profile sexual misconduct media triggers sex harassment recall and reinterpretation. *Equality, Diversity and Inclusion: An International Journal, 39*(1), 68–86. https://doi.org/10.1108/EDI-12-2018-0222

APPG. (2021). *The prevalence and reporting of sexual harassment in UK public spaces: A report by the APPG for UN women*. https://www.unwomenuk.org/site/wp-content/uploads/2021/03/APPG-UN-Women-Sexual-Harassment-Report_Updated.pdf

Armstrong, E. A., Gleckman-Krut, M., & Johnson, L. (2018). Silence, power, and inequality: An intersectional approach to sexual violence. *Annual Review of Sociology, 44*, 99–122.

Baroness Casey of Blackstock. (2023). *An independent review into the standards or behaviour and internal culture of the metropolitan police service*. https://www.met.police.uk/SysSiteAssets/media/downloads/met/about-us/baroness-casey-review/update-march-2023/baroness-casey-review-march-2023.pdf

Basile, K. C., Breiding, M. J., & Smith, S. G. (2016). Disability and risk of recent sexual violence in the United States. *American Journal of Public Health, 106*(5), 928–933. https://doi.org/10.2105/AJPH.2015.303004.

Bonnan-White, J., Hetzel-Riggin, M. D., Diamond-Welch, B. K., & Tollini, C. (2018). "You blame me, therefore I blame me": The importance of first disclosure partner responses on trauma-related cognitions and distress.

Journal of Interpersonal Violence, 33(8), 1260–1286. https://doi.org/10.1177/0886260515615141.

Brennan, E., & McElvaney, R. (2020). What helps children tell? A qualitative meta-analysis of child sexual abuse disclosure. *Child Abuse Review, 29*(2), 97–113. https://doi.org/10.1002/car.2617.

Bronfenbrenner, U. (1979). *The ecology of human development: Experiments by nature and design.* Harvard University Press.

Buchanan, N. T., Settles, I. H., Hall, A. T., & O'Connor, R. C. (2014). A review of organizational strategies for reducing sexual harassment: Insights from the U. S. military. *Journal of Social Issues, 70*(4), 687–702. https://doi.org/10.1111/josi.12086.

Burton, C. W., & Guidry, J. D. (2021). Reporting intimate partner violence and sexual assault: A mixed methods study of concerns and considerations among college women of color. *Journal of Transcultural Nursing, 32*(4), 370–381. https://doi.org/10.1177/1043659620941583.

Campbell, R. (2008). The psychological impact of rape victims. *American Psychologist, 63*(8), 702.

Collins, P. H. (2017). On violence, intersectionality and transversal politics. *Ethnic and Racial Studies, 40*(9), 1460–1473. https://doi.org/10.1080/01419870.2017.1317827.

Combes, G., Damery, S., Gunby, C., Harlock, J., Isham, L., et al. (2019). Supporting survivors of sexual violence: Protocol for a mixed-methods, co-research study of the role, funding and commissioning of specialist services provided by the voluntary sector in England. *British Medical Journal Open, 9*(12), Article e035739. https://doi.org/10.1136/bmjopen-2019-035739

Committee on the Impacts of Sexual Harassment in Academia. (2018). *Sexual harassment of women: Climate, culture, and consequences in academic sciences, engineering, and medicine* (p. 24994). National Academies Press. https://doi.org/10.17226/24994.

Cossar, J., Belderson, P., & Brandon, M. (2019). Recognition, telling and getting help with abuse and neglect: Young people's perspectives. *Children and Youth Services Review, 106*, 104469. https://doi.org/10.1016/j.childyouth.2019.104469.

Cox, B., Jewitt, C., & MacIver, E. (2023). *Surviving healthcare: Sexual violence in the healthcare workforce.* Survivor in Scrubs. https://www.survivinginscrubs.co.uk/app/uploads/2023/11/Surviving-in-Scrubs-Surviving-Healthcare-Report.pdf

de Souza Costa, Y. R., Lavorato, S. N., & de Campos Baldin, J. J. C. M. (2020). Violence against women and drug-facilitated sexual assault (DFSA):

A review of the main drugs. *Journal of Forensic and Legal Medicine, 74*, 102020. https://doi.org/10.1016/j.jflm.2020.102020

Du Mont, J., & White, D. (2007). *The uses and impacts of medico-legal evidence in sexual assault cases: A global review*. WHO. https://apps.who.int/iris/bitstream/handle/10665/43795/9789241596046_eng.pdf

EVAW alliance. (2022). *Violence against women and girls (VAWG) code of practice*. https://www.endviolenceagainstwomen.org.uk/wp-content/uploads/2022/05/VAWG-Code-of-Practice-16.05.22-Final.pdf

Fritz, N., Malic, V., Paul, B., & Zhou, Y. (2021). Worse than objects: The depiction of black women and men and their sexual relationship in pornography. *Gender Issues, 38*(1), 100–120.

Hagemann-White, C., Kavemann, B., Heinz, K., Meysen, T., Puchert, R. et al. (2010). Factors at play in the perpetration of violence against women, violence against children and sexual orientation violence-a multi-level interactive model. *European Commission*. https://www.humanconsultancy.com/assets/understanding-perpetration/understanding-perpetration.html

Heeks, M., Reed, S., Tafsiri, M., & Prince, S. (2018). *The economic and social costs of crime second edition*. Home Office. https://assets.publishing.service.gov.uk/government/uploads/system/uploads/attachment_data/file/732110/the-economic-and-social-costs-of-crime-horr99.pdf

Heilman, B., & Barker, G. (2018). *Masculine norms and violence: Making the connections*. Promundo-US. https://promundoglobal.org/wp-content/uploads/2018/04/Masculine-Norms-and-Violence-Making-the-Connection-20180424.pdf

Herlihy, J., & Turner, S. (2015). Untested assumptions: Psychological research and credibility assessment in legal decision-making. *European Journal of Psychotraumatology, 6*(1), 27380. https://doi.org/10.3402/ejpt.v6.27380.

Hester, M., & Lilley, S. J. (2017). Rape investigation and attrition in acquaintance, domestic violence and historical rape cases. *Journal of Investigative Psychology and Offender Profiling, 14*(2), 175–188. https://doi.org/10.1002/jip.1469.

Higson-Sweeney, N., & Meyrick, J. (2022). "Who could help me? There was nothing. I brought it on myself": A qualitative study exploring UK university student experiences of sexual violence. *PsyPAG Quarterley, 122.*

HM Government. (2021). *The end-to-end rape review report on findings and actions* (p. 68). https://assets.publishing.service.gov.uk/government/uploads/system/uploads/attachment_data/file/994816/end-to-end-rape-review-report.pdf

HMICFRS. (2021). *Rape monitoring group force summaries 2019/20*. Accessed March 20, 2023, https://www.justiceinspectorates.gov.uk/hmicfrs/police-forces/data/rape-monitoring-group/rape-monitoring-group-dashboard-summaries/rape-monitoring-group-force-summaries/

Hohl, K., & Stanko, E. A. (2024). *Policing rape: The way forward*. Routledge. Accessed April 9, 2024, https://www.taylorfrancis.com/books/mono/10.4324/9780429444869/policing-rape-katrin-hohl-elizabeth-stanko

Home Affairs Committee. (2024). Non contact sexual offences, oral evidence Clare McGlynn. *HC 504*. https://committees.parliament.uk/oralevidence/14324/pdf/

Hooper, L., & Meyrick, J. (2025). Trauma has an echo: A mixed methods study exploring barriers to routine healthcare for survivors of sexual violence in a UK higher education setting. *BMJ Open, 15*(5), e102181. https://doi.org/10.1136/bmjopen-2025-102181

Hudspeth, N., Cameron, J., Baloch, S., Tarzia, L., & Hegarty K. (2022). Health practitioners' perceptions of structural barriers to the identification of intimate partner abuse: A qualitative meta-synthesis. *BMC Health Services Research, 22*(1), 96. https://doi.org/10.1186/s12913-022-07491-8.

Hudspith, L. F., Wages, N., Willmott, D., & Gallagher B. (2023). Forty years of rape myth acceptance interventions: A systematic review of what works in naturalistic institutional settings and how this can be applied to educational guidance for jurors. *Trauma, Violence, & Abuse, 24*(2), 981–1000. https://doi.org/10.1177/15248380211050575.

Jaffe, A. E., DiLillo, D., Hoffman, L., Haikalis, M., & Dykstra, R. E. (2015). Does it hurt to ask? A meta-analysis of participant reactions to trauma research. *Clinical Psychology Review, 40*, 40–56. https://doi.org/10.1016/j.cpr.2015.05.004.

Jakubowski, K. P., Murray, V., Stokes, N., & Thurston, C. (2021). Sexual violence and cardiovascular disease risk: A systematic review and meta-analysis. *Maturitas, 153*, 48–60. https://doi.org/10.1016/j.maturitas.2021.07.014.

Lanier, M. (2010). Epidemiological criminology (EpiCrim): Definition and application. *Journal of Theoretical and Philosophical Criminology, 2*(1), 63–103.

Lanthier, S., Du Mont, J., & Mason, R. (2018). Responding to delayed disclosure of sexual assault in health settings: A systematic review. *Trauma, Violence, & Abuse, 19*(3), 251–265.

Lemaigre, C., Taylor, E. P., & Gittoes, C. (2017). Barriers and facilitators to disclosing sexual abuse in childhood and adolescence: A systematic review.

Child Abuse & Neglect, 70, 39–52. https://doi.org/10.1016/j.chiabu.2017.05.009.

Lomax, J., & Meyrick, J. (2020). Systematic review: Effectiveness of psychosocial interventions on wellbeing outcomes for adolescent or adult victim/survivors of recent rape or sexual assault. *Journal of health psychology*, 1359105320950799.

Lorimer, K., Greco, G., & Lorgelly, P. (2023). A new sexual wellbeing paradigm grounded in capability approach concepts of human flourishing and social justice. *Culture, Health & Sexuality, 25*(10), 1402–1417. https://doi.org/10.1080/13691058.2022.2158236.

McCormack, D., Subburamu, S., Guzman, G., Carmen C., Darapanemi, R., Lis, R., Sima, N., Sperling, J., & Corbo, J. (2022). Traumatic injuries in sexual assault patients in the emergency department. *Western Journal of Emergency Medicine, 23*(5), 672–677. https://doi.org/10.5811/westjem.2022.1.53994.

McElvaney, R. (2019). Helping children to tell about their experiences of sexual abuse. *Child Abuse Review, 28*(2), 166–172. https://doi.org/10.1002/car.2559.

McElvaney, R., Greene, S., & Hogan, D. (2012). Containing the secret of child sexual abuse. *Journal of Interpersonal Violence, 27*(6), 1155–1175. https://doi.org/10.1177/0886260511424503.

McGlynn, P. C. (2022). *Challenging anti-carceral feminism: Criminalisation, justice and continuum thinking*. https://doi.org/10.2139/ssrn.4132898.

McGuffey, C. S. (2013). Rape and racial appraisals: Culture, intersectionality, and black women's accounts of sexual assault. *Du Bois Review: Social Science Research on Race, 10*(1), 109–130. https://doi.org/10.1017/S1742058X12000355

Meltzer, C. E. (2023). Isolated incidents. Media reporting on violence against women in the German press. *Journalism Practice, 0*(0), 1–20. https://doi.org/10.1080/17512786.2022.2162952.

Meyrick, J. (2022). *#metoo for women and men: Understanding power through sexual harassment*. Routledge. Accessed June 16, 2022, https://www.routledge.com/MeToo-for-Women-and-Men-Understanding-Power-through-Sexual-Harassment/Meyrick/p/book/9780367767976

Meyrick, J., & Anning, A. (2021). *It's about getting your life back: Evaluation of justice groups*. University of the West of England. Unpublished.

Meyrick, J., Adams, R., & Cutland, M. (2023). Co-produced patient pathway for sexual health follow-up with children and young people using a paediatric sexual assault referral centre (SARC): facilitating elements of self-care and self-testing. *BMJ Sexual & Reproductive Health* [Preprint]. https://doi.org/10.1136/bmjsrh-2023-201866.

Meyrick, J., Bennett, A., & McGovern, K. M. (2024a). Sexual and domestic violence and abuse: Asking and telling in sexual health services. In *STI & HIV 2023 World Congress*.

Meyrick, J., McCartan, K., Eason, A., Curtis, B., & Rees, E. (2024b). Across landscapes and lifetimes: Causes and solutions of gender-based violence from survivors of violence against women and girls (VAWG). *Journal of Sexual Aggression* [Preprint].

Miller, C. J., Adjognon, O. L., Brady, J. E., Dichter, M. E., & Iverson, K. M. (2021). Screening for intimate partner violence in healthcare settings: An implementation-oriented systematic review. *Implementation Research and Practice, 2*, 26334895211039894. https://doi.org/10.1177/26334895211039894.

Mullany, L., & Trickett, L. (2018). *Misogyny hate crime evaluation report*. https://www.nottingham.ac.uk/lipp/documents/misogyny-evaluation-report.pdf

O'Doherty, L., Whelan, M., Carter, G. J., Brown, K., Tarzia, L., Hegarty, K., Feder, G., & Brown, D. J. (2023). Psychosocial interventions for survivors of rape and sexual assault experienced during adulthood. *Cochrane Database of Systematic Reviews [Preprint], 10*. https://doi.org/10.1002/14651858.CD013456.pub2.

Office for National Statistics. (2024). *Estimates of the population for the UK, England, Wales, Scotland, and Northern Ireland: Mid-year population estimates, UK, June 2020*. Accessed August, 8 2024, https://www.ons.gov.uk/peoplepopulationandcommunity/populationandmigration/populationestimates/datasets/populationestimatesforukenglandandwalesscotlandandnorthernireland

Office for National Statistics. (2021a). *Sexual offences in England and Wales overview: Year ending March 2020*. Accessed February 4, 2022, https://www.ons.gov.uk/peoplepopulationandcommunity/crimeandjustice/bulletins/sexualoffencesinenglandandwalesoverview/march2020

Office for National Statistics. (2021b). *Sexual offences prevalence and victim characteristics, England and Wales: Year ending March 2020—Appendix Tables: 'Table 1: Prevalence of sexual assault among adults aged 16 to 74, by type of sexual assault and sex, year ending March 2020'*. Accessed February 4, 2022, https://www.ons.gov.uk/peoplepopulationandcommunity/crimeandjustice/datasets/sexualoffencesprevalenceandvictimcharacteristicsenglandandwales

Office for National Statistics. (2021c). *Nature of sexual assault by rape or penetration, England and Wales: Year ending March 2020.* Accessed November 10, 2021, https://www.ons.gov.uk/peoplepopulationandcommunity/crimeandjustice/articles/natureofsexualassaultbyrapeorpenetrationenglandandwales/yearendingmarch2020

Orchowski, L. M., & Gidycz, C. A. (2012). To whom do college women confide following sexual assault? A prospective study of predictors of sexual assault disclosure and social reactions. *Violence against Women, 18*(3), 264–288.

Peter-Hagene, L. C., & Ullman, S. E. (2018). Longitudinal effects of sexual assault victims' drinking and self-blame on posttraumatic stress disorder. *Journal of Interpersonal Violence, 33*(1), 83–93. https://doi.org/10.1177/0886260516636394.

Pugh, B., & Becker, P. (2018). Exploring definitions and prevalence of verbal sexual coercion and its relationship to consent to unwanted sex: Implications for affirmative consent standards on college campuses. *Behavioral Sciences, 8*(8), 69. https://doi.org/10.3390/bs8080069

Recalde-Esnoz, I., Prego-Meleiro, P., Montalvo, G., & Del Castillo, H. (2024). Drug-facilitated sexual assault: A systematic review. *Trauma, Violence, & Abuse, 25*(3), 1814–1825.

Reed, R. A., Pamlanye, J. T., Truex, H. R., Murphy-Neilson, M. C., Kunaniec, K. P., Newins, A. R., & Wilson, L. C. (2020). Higher rates of unacknowledged rape among men: The role of rape myth acceptance. *Psychology of Men & Masculinities, 21*(1), 162.

Richie, B. E. (2012). *Arrested justice: Black women, violence, and America's prison nation.* New York University Press. https://doi.org/10.18574/nyu/9780814723913.001.0001.

Rivara, F., Adhia, A., Lyons, V., Massey, A., Mills, B., Morgan, E., Simckes, M., & Rowhani-Rahbar, A. (2019). The effects of violence on health. *Health Affairs, 38*(10), 1622–1629. https://doi.org/10.1377/hlthaff.2019.00480.

Schwarz, J., Gibson, S., & Lewis-Arévalo, C. (2017). Sexual assault on college campuses: Substance use, victim status awareness, and barriers to reporting. *Building Healthy Academic Communities Journal, 1*(2), 45–60.

Sen, P., Borges, U., Guallar, E., & Cochran J. (2018). Towards an end to sexual harassment: The urgency and nature of change in the era of #metoo. *UN Women.* https://www.unwomen.org/en/digital-library/publications/2018/11/towards-an-end-to-sexual-harassment#view

Sigurdardottir, S., & Halldorsdottir, S. (2021). Persistent suffering: The serious consequences of sexual violence against women and girls, their search for inner healing and the significance of the #metoo movement. *International Journal of Environmental Research and Public Health, 18*(4), 1849. https://doi.org/10.3390/ijerph18041849.

Slatton, B. C., & Richard, A. L. (2020). Black women's experiences of sexual assault and disclosure: Insights from the margins. *Sociology Compass, 14*(6), e12792. https://doi.org/10.1111/soc4.12792.

Spotting the Signs. (2023). BASHH + Brook. https://www.brook.org.uk/spotting-the-signs-tool/

Stensvehagen, M. T., Bronken, B. A., Lien, L., & Larsson, G. (2023). Association of daily hassles, daily uplifts, coping styles and stress-related symptoms among women exposed to sexual abuse—A cross-sectional study. *Scandinavian Journal of Caring Sciences, 37*(1), 117–130. https://doi.org/10.1111/scs.13107.

Tillewein, H., Shokeen, N., Powers, P., Sanchez, A. J. R., Sandles-Palmer, S., & Desjarlais, K. (2023). Silencing the rainbow: Prevalence of LGBTQ+ students who do not report sexual violence. *International Journal of Environmental Research and Public Health, 20*(3), 2020. https://doi.org/10.3390/ijerph20032020.

Towl, G. J., & Walker, T. (2019). *Tackling sexual violence at universities: An international perspective*. Routledge.

Ullman, S. E., Foynes, M. M., & Tang, S. S. S. (2010). *Benefits and barriers to disclosing sexual trauma: A contextual approach*. Taylor & Francis.

Ullman, S. E., & Peter-Hagene, L. (2014). Social reactions to sexual assault disclosure, coping, perceived control, and PTSD symptoms in sexual assault victims. *Journal of Community Psychology, 42*(4), 495–508. https://doi.org/10.1002/jcop.21624

Ungar, M., Tutty, L. M., McConnell, S., Barter, K., & Fairholm, J. (2009). What Canadian youth tell us about disclosing abuse. *Child Abuse & Neglect, 33*(10), 699–708. https://doi.org/10.1016/j.chiabu.2009.05.002.

Van der Kolk, B. A. (1994). The body keeps the score: Memory and the evolving psychobiology of posttraumatic stress. *Harvard Review of Psychiatry, 1*(5), 253–265. https://doi.org/10.3109/10673229409017088.

Walfield, S. M. (2021). "Men cannot be raped": Correlates of male rape myth acceptance. *Journal of Interpersonal Violence, 36*(13–14), 6391–6417. https://doi.org/10.1177/0886260518817777.

Wang, Y. X., Sun, Y., Missmer, S. A., Rexrode, K. M., Roberts, A. L., Chavarro, J. E., & Rich-Edwards, J. W. (2023). Association of early life physical and sexual abuse with premature mortality among female nurses: Prospective cohort study. *BMJ*, 381, e073613. https://doi.org/10.1136/bmj-2022-073613.

Wilson, L. C., & Miller, K. E. (2016). Meta-analysis of the prevalence of unacknowledged rape. *Trauma, Violence, & Abuse, 17*(2), 149–159. https://doi.org/10.1177/1524838015576391.

Zinzow, H. M., & Thompson, M. (2011). Barriers to reporting sexual victimization: Prevalence and correlates among undergraduate women. *Journal of Aggression, Maltreatment & Trauma, 20*(7), 711–725.

Part III

Treatment and Rehabilitation

8

The Nature of Trauma-Informed Practice in Work with Men Convicted of a Sexual Offence

Chris Pawson, Sarah Senker, and Anne Eason

Introduction

Several theoretical frameworks concerning the rehabilitation of those convicted of a sexual offence have drawn the distinction between static and dynamic risk factors (Bonta & Andrews, 2017) including the risk-need responsivity model (Andrews & Bonta, 2010). Static factors are conceptualised as predictors of reoffending that tend to be historical; perceived as unchangeable, and outside the scope of intervention, e.g. age at first offence (Grieger & Hosser, 2014). Conversely, dynamic factors can be addressed and their risk ameliorated during treatment or rehabilitation, e.g. substance abuse, criminal network or mental health factors (Bonta et al., 2014; Wooditch et al., 2014). According to such models therefore, the effort of those involved in treatment, rehabilitation and post-release monitoring is proposed to be best deployed attending to

C. Pawson (✉) · S. Senker · A. Eason
University of the West of England, Bristol, UK
e-mail: chris.pawson@uwe.ac.uk

K. McCartan et al. (eds.), *Developing and Implementing a Public Health and Criminological Approach to Tackling Sexual Abuse*, Palgrave Studies in Risk, Crime and Society, https://doi.org/10.1007/978-3-031-93634-0_8

dynamic factors (Bonta & Andrews, 2017). However, the current authors propose that this risks the potential creation of a 'blind-spot' in applied rehabilitative practice. Features of the offender's past that might traditionally be thought of as static, should be reconsidered based on their potential to exert sustained and persistent influence on current behaviour and future risk of recidivism. We argue that features of the developmental history of offenders, such as abuse history and trauma exert precisely this persistent influence, and ought to be appraised as dynamic, and prioritised, within the scope of intervention, treatment, and support.

Within an epidemiological criminology framework (McCartan & Kemshall, 2023) an understanding of the offender requires an understanding of their broad range of interactions and experiences. This includes those from across the life course and those that may, for a range of reasons, be relatively unacknowledged and / or inaccessible, e.g. offenders' own experiences as victims. Despite the prevalence of work on adverse childhood experiences (ACES), victimhood as a criminogenic factor has traditionally been frequently neglected in research (Funk, 1999). Until recently, acknowledgment of victimhood and associated trauma has rarely been acknowledged and integrated within applied preventative work with offenders (Grady et al., 2022; Lewis et al., 2019). One of the reasons for this may be a relative lack of robust theorisation, theoretical testing, and effective evaluation of applied work with trauma—particularly with those convicted of sexual offences (Heffernen & Ward, 2020; Jones, 2020). However, in the case of the relationship between traumatic victimisation and sexual offending behaviour the current authors argue that there may be several additional reasons why neglect may persist at both theoretical and applied levels. These relate specifically to the nature of trauma, but also the complexities, demands and implications of acknowledging and addressing its significance in the lives of offenders (by both practitioners and those convicted of crimes).

In this chapter, we argue that trauma and its significance for work with victim-offenders[1] may be particularly under-acknowledged for a number

[1] The authors use the term victim-offender to denote those convicted of a sexual offence who have themselves been subjected to previous trauma including but not limited to abuse.

of reasons, including the offender being unable to voice traumatic experience due to the psychological distress that recall can cause; perhaps due to fear of the societal stigmatisation that comes with disclosure of these experiences or the possibility of elevated risk assessment leading to further lifestyle restrictions. The possibility also exists that even if the offender voices these experiences, the criminal justice system and wider society may not be open to hearing or understanding it. Trauma experienced by the offender is not considered in the Risk of Serious Harm Guidance (Public Protection Group, 2020) and thus may not be identified as crucial to harm reduction. We ask, are systemic and societal perceptions sufficiently liberated from the victim-offender dichotomy to meaningfully work with trauma as a dynamic risk factor? The authors argue that at best this dichotomy remains sufficiently pervasive that acknowledgment of any victim-offender overlap is controversial. At worst, it may entirely prohibit acknowledging the potential psychological distress of offenders—let alone compassionately attend to it. As long as victimhood and potential associated trauma histories of offenders remain subjugated, then the application of the epidemiological criminology (EpiCrim) model is undermined. More specifically, if these broader developmental or life course (chronosystemic) factors (e.g. adverse childhood experience and trauma) are not considered or routinely addressed, then the explanatory potential of the socio-ecological model is compromised, and the preventative utility of the EpiCrim approach to sexual offending cannot be fully realised.

What is Trauma?

Intense affective experience during adverse events can have a long-standing psychological and physiological impact on the individual. These impacts can result from single events, or from repetitive and sustained experiences of adversity that leave the individual feeling unsafe. Furthermore, when the psychological impact of these events and the perceived threat and lack of safety is experienced as overwhelming to the individual, then this is described as trauma. Importantly, it is the subjective interpretation of the threat that can lead to overwhelm, rather than any objective level of threat. Therefore, traumatic events and how they are interpreted and experienced are unique—and therefore so too are the effects. However, in response to overwhelming (traumatic) events, there are a number of outcomes (trauma responses) that are frequently observed. Physiologically, the arousal and underlying cortico-limbic systems are altered which can give rise to reactions such as sleep and appetite disturbance, elevated cortisol, hyperarousal, and persistent fatigue (Murphy et al., 2022). The initiation of a conditioned fear response can also give rise to intrusive memories and longer-term alterations in cognitive appraisal, including hypervigilance and generalisations of perceived danger (Foa et al., 1999). In psychological terms, this can manifest as difficulties in regulating affective responses, and ultimately result in hostility, anxiety, and depression. Emotional dysregulation associated with trauma can be particularly pervasive for those experiencing traumatic events during childhood (van der Kolk et al., 1993), and with this there is a risk of impaired regulation of trauma-related impulses and maladaptive behaviour (Mills & Teeson, 2019).

In short, the neuropsychological impact and emotion regulation issues associated with traumatic experiences are likely to be particularly salient in terms of risk of recidivism. So too will emotional numbing, the normalisation of the experience of abuse, and substance use—all of which are frequently deployed as a means of coping with trauma and abuse (Briggs & Hawkins, 1996; Ford et al., 2013; McMackin et al., 2002; Orsillo et al., 2007; Turner & Rettenberger, 2020).

Trauma and Sexual Offending: Prevalence

Research has found that females are more likely to be subjected to sexual abuse, and female survivors of child sexual abuse (CSA) are more likely to experience greater trauma in the context of abuse. However, the prevalence of trauma in the backgrounds of men who offend sexually is increasingly recognised (DeLisi et al., 2014; Jones, 2022). Furthermore, there is significant evidence linking experience of CSA (which is recognised to be a source of trauma), to subsequent sexual offending behaviour (Levenson et al., 2016; Plummer & Cossins, 2018). Ogloff et al. (2012)

found that 5% of male victims of CSA were subsequently convicted of a sexual offence, rising to 9.2% being convicted of sexual offending amongst those abused at the age of 12 years or older. Levenson et al. (2016) found that amongst a population of males convicted of sexual offences the rate of CSA was approximately 14 times that found in the general population.

It is particularly noteworthy that several features that are associated with traumatic abuse (i.e. forms of abuse that are reported as contributing to trauma responses) are the same features of abuse that are associated with increased likelihood of male survivors going on to become abusers themselves. These include increased frequency and severity of abuse, as well as the experience of powerlessness or dependency on the perpetrator (Plummer & Cossins, 2018).

Unresolved Trauma and Recidivism Risk

Despite the increasing evidence concerning the prevalence of adverse childhood experiences such as maltreatment and abuse in the histories of offenders (Grady et al., 2017, 2021), there is still considerable debate surrounding the mechanism underpinning this relationship (Malvaso et al., 2022). Some have proposed social learning processes whereby behaviours perpetrated against victims are then reproduced by these victims against others, including sexual offending behaviours (e.g. Burton, 2000). Others point to the role of adversity and experience of abuse in the development of poor mental health, which in turn can lead to subsequent substance use and criminality. There is also increasing acknowledgment of the potential intersection of victims' trauma in explaining their subsequent offending behaviour (DeLisi et al., 2018; Fox et al., 2015). In other words, a range of features or vulnerabilities co-occur and can also result in a compounding of traumatic response.

Some theorists have proposed that one causal mechanism is that traumatic experience may lead to re-enactment of traumatic experience. Intrusive thoughts concerning previous traumatic sexual experiences drive a preoccupation and need to act out compulsively (Jones, 2022; Van der Kolk, 2014). In terms of sexual offending specifically, Jones

(2022) concludes that "a significant proportion of the antecedent drivers for sexual offending are trauma-linked' (p. 226). This is a conclusion echoed in the accounts of those convicted of sexual offences, who perceive a strong connection between their own experiences as victims and their subsequent offending behaviour (Grady et al., 2022). Furthermore, there is some limited evidence to suggest that there may be value in attending to the processing of trauma in reducing recidivism (Ricci & Clayton, 2016; Wright & Warner, 2020; Wright et al., 2023).

Despite the emerging data suggesting a link between traumatisation and future offending, this has not translated into trauma being readily acknowledged within the criminal justice sector. However, nor does it necessarily mean that all offenders with a trauma history will benefit by talking about their traumatic experience(s). There is evidence that survivors will cope in different ways, and for some it will not be beneficial to express their emotions or discuss their trauma (SAMHSA, 2014). Indeed, Greenwald (2009) notes the significant obstacles many victim-offenders convicted of sexual offences will experience, and the significant potential for harm in facing traumatic memories. Even for those who may benefit, it is also very important to note that victim-offenders may have experienced significant difficulties in previous disclosure, e.g. due to fears concerning accusations or labelling (Watkins & Bentovim, 1992), particularly by those working in the criminal justice system. Furthermore, an additional barrier to disclosure and therapeutic discussions of trauma, is that historically there have also been signals from criminal justice professionals that discussion of adverse childhood experiences and abuse histories should be challenged or avoided (Hindman & Peters, 2001). This has been due to fear of victimisation history either being seen as too easy for offenders to exploit, or it feeding an 'exculpatory' narrative (Jones, 2020) as part of an attempt to rationalise or excuse sexual offending behaviour (Ricci & Clayton, 2016).

Relatedly, and similarly challenging, are the societal signals that 'boys do not get abused' (Paine & Hansen, 2002). This is potentially reinforced by criminology research recognising the role of physical and/or sexual abuse as catalysts for delinquent (and ultimately offending) behaviour, but historically focusing on the significance of this in females (Chesney-Lind, 1997; Holsinger, 1999). A key feature in the context of sexual abuse of males that may result in unprocessed trauma is the increased likelihood of force being involved in males' experiences of CSA (Pierce & Pierce, 1985). Indeed, Burton et al., (2002) specifically postulate that force may be particularly salient in the risk of victimhood that leads to offending behaviour. Connected to this, and a further obstacle to disclosure and processing trauma, is the problem that signals of physiological arousal such as victim erection and ejaculation during abuse can create significant psychological incongruence and discomfort (Bullock & Beckson, 2011). Ultimately, experiences of being abused which included sensations of physical arousal can be confusing and subjectively interpreted as denoting subconscious consent—and therefore become more distressing because they cannot be discussed (Widanaralalage et al., 2022).

What is Trauma-Informed Practice?

Trauma-informed practice (TIP) refers to a way of working that acknowledges the impact of previous negative affective and traumatic experiences in service design and delivery. It has been most prominently seen in work with multiple disadvantage service users (henceforth clients) who frequently require simultaneous support from mental health, substance use, homelessness, and criminal justice services. This is driven by the increasing recognition that these clients often have traumatic experiences in their histories that contribute to the multiple challenges and disadvantages they face (Christensen et al., 2005; Wiewel & Hernandez, 2022).

TIP seeks to work with clients in ways that avoid replicating the interactions, processes and systems that might perpetuate distress, and result in re-traumatisation. Ultimately, this will promote client safety and increase the accessibility of treatment services. The Substance Abuse and Mental Health Services Administration (SAMHSA, 2014) who are frequently cited as informing TIP (including by the U.K. government) conceptualises this way of working as served by six core principles:

Safety (prioritising the physical, psychological and emotional safety of clients and staff)
Trustworthiness (building trust between service users and staff through ensuring transparency when working with service users in terms of an organisation's policies and procedures)
Peer support (ensuring that practice and policy are informed by those with lived experience that is aligned to the experienced of the client)
Collaboration (recognising the value of staff and service user experience in overcoming challenges and working collaboratively to improve the system as a whole)
Empowerment (through sharing power in ways that are responsive to individual need, and give service users and staff a strong voice in decision-making at both individual and organisational level)
Cultural, historical and gender issues (moving beyond stereotypes and biases and acknowledging the intersectionality of, for example, structural inequalities, and historical barriers for some groups)

TIP will often involve specific types of therapeutic practice (see below), but also the training of staff to create climates that can support these principles. Often this will involve introducing the concept of trauma through training and encouraging reflection on what these principles mean for their engagement with clients. This is frequently followed by a review of systems, policies and processes within their organisation or service, often assisted by toolkits aimed at their alignment with key principles (e.g. Homes, 2021).

Trauma-informed Practice with those convicted of a sexual offence: What does it look like?

As well as striving to ensure increased staff awareness of the potential role of trauma in the lives of clients and avoid reproduction of dynamics and triggers that may re-traumatise, TIP is also manifested in specific therapeutic approaches to working with men convicted of sexual offences.

These include specific psychodynamic approaches (Blumenthal et al., 2018; Parker, 2004); models focused on the role of attachment (Grady et al., 2017, 2019), and compassion-focused care (Taylor, 2017). There are also several small-scale trials and case study reports of participant experiences of the use of Eye Movement Desensitisation and Reprocessing (EMDR) with encouraging results (Ricci et al., 2006; Wright & Warner, 2020; Wright et al., 2023). Others have explicitly addressed trauma through the deployment of exposure techniques (Briere, 2019), although this is not without its critics (e.g. Norcross & Wampold, 2019).

As previously noted, working with and processing trauma directly in work with people convicted of sexual offences can be very challenging, and potentially even harmful if the broader environment is not conducive and enforcing of trauma-informed principles (Greenwald, 2009). With that in mind, many approaches avoid direct attempts to process the trauma and its causes, but instead focus on working with the consequences of the trauma. This includes reducing risks associated with emotional dysregulation or substance use. For example, in the 'Enhanced Thinking Skills' programme (Andrews & Bonta, 2010) difficulties with impulse control are approached through the development of cognitive skills for self-regulation. Greenwald (2009) has developed a cognitive behavioural framework aimed at addressing the 'trauma-informed offence cycle'. This approach assumes that maladaptive behaviours are deployed by the victim-offender to cope with trauma-related intrusive thoughts and compulsions. This approach aims to equip the client to recognise and challenge the risky or offending behaviours that they are deploying to ameliorate the discomfort of trauma triggers, e.g. powerlessness. Similar therapeutic principles are described by Jones (2020), but with the incorporation of triggers specifically centred around attachment difficulties. Also, within the stable of cognitively oriented approaches, schema therapy seeks to challenge the offender's cognitive distortions that they feel may justify offending behaviour (Bernstein et al., 2023; Oettingen & Rajtar-Zembaty, 2022). However, in the case of the victim-offender convicted of sexual offences, Grady et al. (2017) have noted the risks of confrontational exchanges during the repeated challenges to cognitions. Grady et al. (2017) also note the importance of ensuring that the challenge is aimed at the underlying maladaptive schema that gave rise to those distortions. In terms of an impact on desistance, trauma-informed approaches that address the prior experiences and cognition underlying offending behaviour are likely to be more effective than those merely addressing the behaviours themselves. However, resources and the challenges of delivering ongoing psychological interventions in the prison environment may make symptom- rather than cause-oriented intervention more attractive.

Several scholars in the field have pointed towards the value of more relational and integrative approaches, arguing for the importance of building therapeutic trust (Grady et al., 2019). Given that trauma is related to the overwhelm associated with threats to safety then building trust and a sense of safety seems entirely consistent with likely therapeutic benefits. It also aligns very closely with the principles of trauma-informed practice (SAMHSA, 2014). However, again, there remains a question as to how achievable this is in the context of secure settings including prisons and secure hospitals as well as probation.

An integrated approach that addresses attachment, cognition, self-regulation skills, and their inter-relationships has received recent attention. The Good Lives Model (GLM) is based on the premise that individuals (whether offenders or not) will be seeking to move towards a set of similar states or life goals (Yates & Prescott, 2011). However, when challenges in progress towards these goals are experienced, then these goals can be ascertained through anti-social means or offending. Furthermore, trauma can also impede progress, and identifying the ways in which trauma creates challenges can facilitate a meaningful therapeutic journey for the client.

Trauma-informed Practice with Offenders: What are the Barriers?

Some authors have argued that the more relational and integrated approaches to working with men convicted of sexual offences are more aligned with principles of TIP (Levenson et al., 2020). If we assume the principles of GLM are sound, and that addressing trauma will act as an enabler to reduce risk of offending and move towards goals, then treatment approaches that are more trauma-informed should have greater success. With that in mind, it is important to explore how to facilitate greater trauma-informed practice, and one approach is to explore what potential barriers might exist (Senker et al., 2023).

The first challenge is not specific to TIP with offenders, but relates to the importance of shared understandings, and ensuring that researchers and practitioners are all talking about the same thing when referring to trauma and trauma-informed practice. Edleman (2023) notes that the term trauma is often erroneously used to describe the events themselves, rather than the physiological and psychological state created when the individual feels threatened by events and uncontained. Relatedly, and because trauma relates to how the individual constructs their experience, it is important to note that not everyone experiencing adversity will be traumatised. To promote psychological safety and TIP, practitioners need the ability to instil confidence in clients and each other—and therefore accuracy, a shared understanding and language are important.

Even with a shared definition of trauma, there is also variation in definitions of what it is to apply that to engagement in trauma-informed practice. Is attendance at trauma-informed training sufficient, and where is the delineation between therapeutic practice and TIP? These issues are further complicated by emerging nomenclature related to gradations of preparedness for TIP. These include distinctions between being trauma-aware and trauma-informed, and now trauma-enhanced, which are often viewed as bronze, silver, and gold 'standards' which are evaluated by external agencies.

The next, but related challenge, relates to the process of ensuring staff and organisations are adequately trained to work with trauma safely. A key question relates to how to train staff adequately to support them to cope with disclosure of trauma histories. Edelman (2023) provides a salutary warning concerning the training processes in TIP, which frequently openly discuss trauma but fail to consider whether staff trainees may have their own trauma histories and triggers. There is a significant literature on the psychological impact of working with those who have experienced trauma, and the potential for what is variously described as 'secondary' or 'vicarious' trauma (Chouliara et al., 2009; McNeillie & Rose, 2021). Edelman points to several examples where assumptions and a lack of adequate trigger warnings can at best leave staff closed down and disengaged from training, but at worst closed down and traumatised.

Engagement with training is important to ensure shared understandings, but also to ensure that staff are adequately prepared for the trauma histories that might be shared with them after training and on the job. Furthermore, even if they have the sufficient skills to support themselves and contain the client, it is important to consider whether they are sufficiently supported in terms of time and physical resources. Given the frequent resource constraints in the prison service, even compassionate and dedicated staff may find themselves confronted with stress and burnout (see Chapter 10) that make it more difficult for them to 'model the TIP model'. To cultivate the relationships and psychological climate to enable trust and containment, staff need significant psychological resource, including opportunities for debriefing and reflective practice.

To be truly trauma-informed in practice demands not just training, skills and support of individual staff, but also requires an analysis of organisational climate, practice, and policy. TIP is not a 'one off' review, nor a checklist for one *part* of an organisation. It is integrated, holistic, and longitudinal. Therapeutic sessions can be trauma-informed and very supportive of the individual client, but this is of limited utility if the client then leaves a therapy session or intervention and has to endure interactions and environments in which they experience abuse from others in prison, or power differentials in interactions with staff. Prescott (2020) notes that the professional roles and boundaries of those within secure settings can be particularly blurry. He notes that interactions between staff and clients can frequently be characterised by a judgmental tone and be experienced as disempowering for the client. Relatedly, Senker et al. (2023) ask whether the physical environment of prisons and their design based on managing risk, can ever truly support trauma-informed practice even if individuals on the front-line are minded implementing this.

Conclusion

In conclusion, where experiences of abuse that result in trauma are part of the histories of those convicted of sexual offences, these experiences should not be ignored. These experiences are frequently associated with offending behaviour and act as a dynamic, rather than static risk factor. We argue that if left unaddressed, these experiences can hinder long lasting rehabilitation and thwart desistance, disenabling recovery and risking consequent harmful behaviour. Trauma-informed practice seeks to acknowledge the impact of trauma on the neurology, physiology, and psychology of the individual. It explicitly recognises that trauma can manifest cognitively and behaviourally, including playing a part in initiating and maintaining offending behaviour. Furthermore, TIP seeks to create interventions and environments that are accessible, and which avoid recreating the dynamics that serve as triggers or propagate trauma. It is through the delivery of these principles, that TIP can support positive recovery and the development of empathy, self-regulation and positive community integration.

In terms of realising the potential of the EpiCrim model, and developing primary and secondary prevention strategies, the authors argue TIP is essential. It is only by adopting a life course perspective and acknowledging developmental risk factors, that risk can be effectively ameliorated. However, as has also been argued in this chapter, TIP working with men convicted of sexual offences, and particularly when the work is undertaken within the confines of the criminal justice system, is not without challenges. This is a result of the stigmatisation these individuals face relating to their particular offending; challenges in moving from pathologisation to compassion, the difficulty in viewing individuals as experiencing trauma themselves *and* harming others, and the organisational barriers associated with a system that prioritises risk of harm reduction and public protection. It is hoped that in highlighting the importance of a life course developmental approach that acknowledges trauma, and therefore the value of TIP (and its challenges), this can contribute to the ongoing discussions around the EpiCrim approach—and its contribution to the reduction of offending and sexually harmful behaviour.

References

Andrews, D. A., & Bonta, J. A. (2010). *The psychology of criminal conduct* (5th ed.). Anderson.

Bernstein, D. P., Keulen-de Vos, M., Clercx, M., de Vogel, V., Kersten, G. C. M., Lancel, M., Jonkers, P. P., Bogaerts, S., Slaats, M., Broers, N. J., Deenen, T. A. M., & Arntz, A. (2023). Schema therapy for violent PD offenders: A randomized clinical trial. *Psychological Medicine, 53*(1), 88–102. https://doi.org/10.1017/s0033291721001161

Blumenthal, S., Wood, H., & Williams, A. (2018). *Assessing risk: A relational approach.* Routledge.

Bonta, J., & Andrews, D. A. (2017). *The psychology of criminal conduct* (6th ed.). Routledge.

Bonta, J., Law, M., & Hanson, R. K. (1998). The prediction of criminal and violent recidivism among mentally disordered offenders: A meta-analysis. *Psychological Bulletin, 39*, 127–144.

Bonta, J., Blais, J., & Wilson, H. A. (2014). A theoretically informed meta-analysis of the risk for general and violent recidivism for mentally disordered offenders. *Aggression and violent behavior, 19*(3), 278-287.

Briere, J. (2019). *Treating risky and compulsive behavior in trauma survivors.* Guilford.

Briggs, F., & Hawkins, R. M. (1996). A comparison of the childhood experiences of convicted male child molesters and men who were sexually abused in childhood and claimed to be nonoffenders. *Child abuse & neglect, 20*(3), 221–233. https://doi.org/10.1016/S0145-2134(95)00145-X

Bullock, C. M., & Beckson, M. (2011). Male victims of sexual assault: Phenomenology, psychology, physiology. *Journal of the American Academy of Psychiatry and the Law Online, 39*(2), 197–205.

Burton, D. L. (2000). Were adolescent sexual offenders children with sexual behavior problems? *Sexual Abuse: A journal of Research and Treatment, 12*(1), 37–48.

Burton, D., Miller, D., & Shill, C. (2002). A social learning theory comparison of the sexual victimization of adolescent sexual offen and nonsexual offending male delinquents. *Child Abuse and Neglect, 26*, 893–907. https://doi.org/10.1016/s0145-2134(02)00360-5

Chesney-Lind, M. (1997). *The female offender*. Sage.

Chouliara, Z., Hutchison, C., & Karatzias, T. (2009). Vicarious traumatisation in practitioners who work with adult survivors of sexual violence and child sexual abuse: Literature review and directions for future research. *Counselling and Psychotherapy Research, 9*(1), 47–56.

Christensen, R. C., Hodgkins, C. C., Garces, L., Estlund, K. L., Miller, M. D., & Touchton, R. (2005). Homeless, mentally ill and addicted: The need for abuse and trauma services. *Journal of Health Care for the Poor and Underserved, 16*(4), 615–622.

DeLisi, M., Fox, B. H., Fully, M., & Vaughn, M. G. (2018). The effects of temperament, psychopathy, and childhood trauma among delinquent youth: A test of DeLisi and Vaughn's temperament-based theory of crime. *International Journal of Law and Psychiatry, 57*, 53–60. https://doi.org/10.1016/j.ijlp.2018.01.006

DeLisi, M., Kosloski, A., Vaughn, M., Caudill, J., & Trulson, C. (2014). Does childhood sexual abuse victimization translate into juvenile sexual offending? New evidence. *Violence, 29*, 620–635. https://doi.org/10.1891/0886-6708.vv-d-13-00003

Edelman, N. (2023). Doing trauma-informed work in a trauma-informed way: Understanding difficulties and finding solutions. *Health Services Insights, 16*, 11786329231215036.

Ford, J. D., Grasso, D. J., Hawke, J., & Chapman, J. F. (2013). Polyvictimization among juvenile justice-involved youths. *Child Abuse and Neglect, 37*(10), 788–800.

Foa, E. B., Ehlers, A., Clark, D. M., Tolin, D. F., & Orsillo, S. M. (1999). The posttraumatic cognitions inventory (PTCI): Development and validation. *Psychological Assessment, 11*(3), 303.

Fox, B. H., Perez, N., Cass, E., Baglivio, M. T., & Epps, N. (2015). Trauma changes everything: Examining the relationship between adverse childhood experiences and serious, violent and chronic juvenile offenders. *Child Abuse and Neglect, 46*, 163–173. https://doi.org/10.1016/j.chiabu.2015.01.011

Funk, S. J. (1999). Risk assessment for juveniles on probation. *Criminal Justice and Behaviour, 26*, 44–68.

Grady, M. D., Levenson, J. S., & Bolder, T. (2017). Linking adverse childhood effects and attachment: A theory of etiology for sexual offending. *Trauma, Violence, and Abuse, 18*(4), 433–444.

Grady, M. D., Levenson, J. S., Glover, J., Kavanagh, S., & Carter, K. (2022). "Hurt people hurt other people": The link between past trauma and sexual offending. *Sexual Offending: Theory, Research, and Prevention, 17*, Article e7361.

Grady, M. D., Looman, J., & Abracen, J. (2019). Childhood abuse, attachment, and psychopathy among individuals who commit sexual offences. *Sexual Addiction and Compulsivity, 26*, 1–26.

Grady, M. D., Yoder, J., & Brown, A. (2021). Childhood maltreatment experiences, attachment, sexual offending: Testing a theory. *Journal of interpersonal violence, 36,* 11–12, NP6183-NP6217.

Greenwald, R. (2009). *Treating problem behaviors: A trauma-informed approach.* Routledge.

Grieger, L., & Hosser, D. (2014). Which risk factors are really predictive? An analysis of Andrews and Bonta's "central eight" risk factors for recidivism in German youth correctional facility inmates. *Criminal Justice and Behavior, 41*(5), 613–634.

Heffernan, R., & Ward, T. (2020). Critical analysis of dynamic risk factors. In *Dynamic risk factors for sexual offending.* SpringerBriefs in Psychology(). Springer. https://doi.org/10.1007/978-3-030-58275-3_2

Hindman, J., & Peters, J. M. (2001). Polygraph testing leads to better understanding adult and juvenile sex offenders. *Federal Probation, 65*(3), 8–15.

Holsinger, K. (1999). *Addressing the distinct experience of the adolescent female: Explaining delinquency and examining the juvenile justice system.* University of Cincinnati.

Homes, A. (2021). *Trauma-informed practice: A toolkit for Scotland*. Scottish Government.

Jones, L. (2020). Trauma, adverse experiences, and offence-paralleling behaviour in the assessment and management of sexual interest. In *Assessing and managing problematic sexual interests* (pp. 251–274). Routledge.

Jones, L. (2022). Trauma and sexual offending: Causal mechanisms and change processes. In *Trauma-informed forensic practice* (pp. 212–230). Routledge.

Levenson, J. S., Willis, G. M., & Prescott, D. S. (2020). Evidence-based practice and the role of trauma-informed care in sex offending treatment. In H. Saby, B. Winder, R. Lievesley, K. Hoken, N. Glagden & P. Banyard (Eds.), *Sexual crime and trauma, sexual crime*. Palgrave Macmillan.

Levenson, J. S., Willis, G., & Prescott, D. S. (2016). Adverse childhood experiences in the lives of male sex offenders and implications for trauma-informed care. *Sexual Abuse a Journal of Research and Treatment, 28*, 340–359.

Lewis, S. J., Arseneault, L., Caspi, A., Fisher, H. L., Matthews, T., Moffitt, T. E., ... & Danese, A. (2019). The epidemiology of trauma and post-traumatic stress disorder in a representative cohort of young people in England and Wales. *The Lancet Psychiatry, 6*(3), 247–256.

Malvaso, C. G., Cale, J., Whitten, T., Day, A., Singh, S., Hackett, L., ... & Ross, S. (2022). Associations between adverse childhood experiences and trauma among young people who offend: A systematic literature review. *Trauma, Violence, and Abuse, 23*(5), 1677–1694.

McCartan, K., & Kemshall, H. (2023). Incorporating quaternary prevention: Understanding the full scope of public health practices in sexual abuse prevention. *International Journal of Offender Therapy and Comparative Criminology, 67*(2–3), 224–246.

McMackin, R. A., Leisen, M. B., Cusack, J. F., LaFratta, J., & Litwin, P. (2002). The relationship of trauma exposure to sex offending behavior among male juvenile offenders. *Journal of Child Sexual Abuse, 11*(2), 25–40.

McNeillie, N., & Rose, J. (2021). Vicarious trauma in therapists: A meta-ethnographic review. *Behavioural and Cognitive Psychotherapy, 49*(4), 426–440.

Mills, K., & Teeson, M. (2019). Trauma-informed care in the context of alcohol and other drug use disorders. In R. Benjamin, J. Haliburn, & S. King (eds) *Humanising mental health care in Australia: A guide to trauma-informed approaches* (pp. 181–194). Routledge.

Murphy, F., Nasa, A., Cullinane, D., Raajakesary, K., Gazzaz, A., Sooknarine, V., ... & Roddy, D. W. (2022). Childhood trauma, the HPA axis and psychiatric illnesses: A targeted literature synthesis. *Frontiers in Psychiatry, 13*, 748372.

Norcross, J. C., & Wamplod, B. E. (2019). Relationships and responsiveness in the psychological treatment of trauma: The tragedy of the APA clinical practice guideline. *Psychotherapy, Theory, Research and Practice, 56*(3), 391–401.

Oettingen, J., & Rajtar-Zembaty, A. (2022). Prospect of using schema therapy in working with sex offenders. *Psychiatria Polska, 56*(6), 1253–1267. https://doi.org/10.12740/pp/143847

Ogloff, J. R. P., Cutajar, M. C., Mann, E., & Mullen, P. (2012). *Child sexual abuse and subsequent offending and victimisation: A 45 year follow-up study (trends and issues in crime and criminal justice no. 440)*. Australian Institute of Criminology.

Orsillo, S. M., Theodore-Oklota, C., Luterek, J. A., & Plumb, J. (2007). The development and psychometric evaluation of the emotional reactivity and numbing scale. *Journal of Nervous and Mental Disease, 195*, 830–836.

Paine, M., & Hansen, D. (2002). Factors influencing children to self sexual abuse. *Clinical Psychology Review, 22*, 271–295. https://doi.org/10.1016/s0272-7358(01)00091-5

Parker, M. (2004). Violence, sexual offending and sexual abuse: Are they linked? A qualitative research study. In D. Jones (Ed.), *Working with dangerous people: The psychotherapy of violence*. Radcliffe Medical Press

Pierce, R., & Pierce, L. (1985). The sexually abused child: A comparison of male and female victims. *Child Abuse and Neglect, 9*, 191–199. https://doi.org/10.1016/0145-2134(85)90011-0

Plummer, M., & Cossins, A. (2018). The cycle of abuse: When victims become offenders. *Trauma, Violence, and Abuse, 19*(3), 286–304.

Public Protection Group. (2020). Risk of Serious Harm Guidance (ROSH). https://assets.publishing.service.gov.uk/media/652cf8c9697260000dccf834/Risk_of_Serious_Harm_Guidance_v3.pdf, Retrieved 25 July 2025.

Prescott, D. S. (2020). Trauma-informed care in secure settings: The whys, hows, and challenges associated. In H. Saby, B. Winder, R. Lievesley, K. Hoken, N. Glagden & P. Banyard (Eds.), *Sexual crime and trauma, sexual crime*. Palgrave Macmillan.

Ricci, R. J., & Clayton, C. A. (2016). EMDR with sex offenders: Using offense drivers to guide conceptualization and treatment. *Journal of EMDR Practice and Research, 10*(2), 104.

Ricci, R. J., Clayton, C. A., & Shapiro, F. (2006). Some effects of EMDR on previously abused child molesters: Theoretical reviews and preliminary findings. *The Journal of Forensic Psychiatry and Psychology, 17*(4), 538–562.

SAMHSA. (2014). SAMHSA's Concept of Trauma and Guidance for a Trauma-Informed Approach. HHS Publication No. (SMA) 14-4884. Substance Abuse and Mental Health Services Administration.

Senker, S., Eason, A., Pawson, C., & McCartan, K. (2023). *Issues, challenges and opportunities for trauma-informed practice*. HMIP Academic Insights 2023/10.

Taylor, J. (2017). Compassion focussed working in secure forensic care. *Journal of Criminological Research, Policy and Practice, 3*, 287–293.

Turner, D., & Rettenberger, M. (2020). Neuropsychological functioning in child sexual abusers: A systematic review. *Aggression and Violent Behavior, 54*, Article 101405.

Van der Kolk, B. (2014). The body keeps the score: Brain, mind, and body in the healing of trauma. *New York, 3*, 14–211.

Van der Kolk, B., Roth, S., Pelcovitz, D., & Mandel, F. (1993). *Complex PTSD: Results of the PTSD field trials for DSM-IV*. American Psychiatric Association.

Watkins, B., & Bentovim, A. (1992). The sexual abuse of male children and adolescents: A review of current research. *Journal of Child Psychology and Psychiatry, 33*, 197–248. https://doi.org/10.1111/j.1469-7610,1992.tb00862.x

Widanaralalage, B. K., Hine, B. A., Murphy, A. D., & Murji, K. (2022). "I didn't feel i was a victim": A phenomenological analysis of the experiences of male-on-male survivors of rape and sexual abuse. *Victims and Offenders, 17*(8), 1147–1172.

Wiewel, B., & Hernandez, L. (2022). Traumatic stress and homelessness: A review of the literature for practitioners. *Clinical Social Work Journal, 50*(2), 218–230.

Wooditch, A., Tang, L. L., & Taxman, F. S. (2014). Which criminogenic need changes are most important in promoting desistance from crime and substance use? *Criminal Justice and Behavior, 41*(3), 276–299.

Wright, L. C., & Warner, A. (2020). EMDR treatment of childhood sexual abuse for a child molester: Self-reported changes in sexual arousal. *Journal of EMDR Practice and Research, 14*(2), 90–103.

Wright, L. C., Palmer, J., Kelly, R., & Derefaka, G. (2023). Eye movement desensitization and reprocessing (EMDR) therapy for childhood sexual abuse memories in men who have sexually offended against children: Changes in perceptions of abuse and offending. *Journal of Forensic Psychology Research and Practice*, 1–19.

Yates, P. M., & Prescott, D. S. (2011). *Building a better life: A good lives model workbook*. Safer Society Press.

Evidence-Based Practice and the Role of Trauma-Informed Care in Sex Offending Treatment SpringerLink

Adverse Childhood Experiences in the Lives of Male Sex Offenders: Implications for Trauma-Informed Care - Jill S. Levenson, Gwenda M. Willis, David S. Prescott, 2016 sagepub.com

"I Couldn't Do It to a Kid Knowing What It Did to Me": The Narratives of Male Sexual Abuse Victims' Resiliency to Sexually Offending PubMed (nih.gov)
Testing the sexually abused-sexual abuser hypothesis: A prospective longitudinal birth cohort study ScienceDirect
https://www.uscourts.gov/fedprob.PDF(ccoso.org)
https://journals.sagepub.com/doi/full/10.1177/1079063214535819

Offending behaviour programmes and interventions

Offending behaviour programmes and interventions GOV.UK(www.gov.uk)
https://assets.publishing.service.gov.uk/media/64085767e90e0740d3cd6fa3/HMPPS_Accredited_Programmes.docx

9

Trauma-Informed Care, Motivational Interviewing, Good Lives, and the Alliance: Putting it All Together in Practice

David S. Prescott

Emily and August

The first time that Emily, a psychotherapist working for the Slate Valley Services, met August was an in interview to determine whether August would be a suitable candidate for that program.[1] August had spent the previous year in a specialized detention program for people determined to need care and supervision by the state (and whom the legal system viewed as needing rehabilitation and not simply incarceration). The case manager for the detention program had worked with August's legal guardian (who was also his father) to determine the best long-term

[1] The example is based on an amalgamation of cases in the author's experience and details altered so that any resemblance to any individual is purely coincidental. Likewise, the various staff members and programs' names are fictitious.

D. S. Prescott (✉)
Safer Society Foundation, Middlebury, VT, USA
e-mail: davidprescott@safersociety.org

K. McCartan et al. (eds.), *Developing and Implementing a Public Health and Criminological Approach to Tackling Sexual Abuse*, Palgrave Studies in Risk, Crime and Society, https://doi.org/10.1007/978-3-031-93634-0_9

placement for him. Such programs could be difficult to find and Slate Valley appeared to be the best option. August's father, the case manager, and Emily all hoped that he would be a good fit for this program.

In the days preceding the interview, Emily had prepared by reading the documentation in August's file. This was always a challenge for Emily, not so much because of the sometimes-graphic offense descriptions, but because of the biased ways that findings were often presented. In one of August's risk assessment reports, the evaluator had used bold text when describing all concerns, yet devoted very little space to August's strengths, positive attributes, hopes, dreams, goals, or aspirations. The result was a risk assessment in the purest sense, highlighting anything risky about August while remaining nearly silent on what programs and providers might do to alleviate those risks.

Likewise, August had been psychiatrically hospitalized, resulting in several diagnoses that might have been apparent in a clinical setting but less evident outside of a hospital environment. Emily's experience was that people like August would sometimes accrue a list of diagnoses that were more related to their functioning within the acutely stressful environment of a compulsory hospitalization than their behavior in the community. For example, various diagnoses related to attention deficits, anxiety, or depression might appear accurate in some ways, but less clear in the context of the origins and etiologies of those conditions. On many occasions, those diagnoses seemed to belie an underlying life narrative of being overwhelmed by adverse early life experiences. Although the diagnoses themselves were not inaccurate, Emily found that helping a client to live in a way less defined by these past events was more effective than thinking of her clients in terms of the criteria of their diagnoses.

On the morning of the interview, Emily prepared herself. To be effective with clients who had sexually abused others and had themselves been traumatized children, Emily was aware that she would have to have knowledge in the areas of:

- normative child and adolescent development
- the impact of trauma at various times in development
- sexual development
- the etiology of mental health difficulties

- the etiology of problematic behaviors
- the principles of effective correctional rehabilitation (including those of risk, need, responsivity; Bonta & Andrews, 2017)

Most importantly, she would need to be able to form an initial working relationship with August, all the while remaining alert to seemingly opposite areas of focus, including:

- the risks he posed
- the treatment needs he evidenced
- his strengths and positive attributes

While keeping each of these in mind, Emily would need to embody the empirically proven characteristics of effective therapists working with individuals who have caused sexual harm. These include being:

- warm
- empathic
- rewarding
- directive (Marshall, 2005)

In preparation for the interview, Emily worked to "get into the mindset of creating new mindsets." This meant that she not only wanted to ask excellent questions and gather information that was not in any reports, but she also wanted to make this the start of any intervention that might follow. Walters et al. (2009) had found that simply going through an alcohol assessment appeared to impact drinking patterns in the months that followed. While no such research exists in the field of treating sexual aggression and offending, she wanted to make sure that her actions paved the way for any work they might do in the future.

The Initial Interview

Emily sat down with August and a staff member named Carol in the living room of the program.

Emily: "How about if we start by you telling me a bit about yourself?"
August: "I'm a sex offender."
Emily (smiling): "And are you other things as well?"
August: "I have to be careful not to offend again for the rest of my life."
Emily: "This sounds like something you've thought a lot about."
August: "I learned it in treatment when I was at that inpatient program back home. Back then, I kind of minimized my behaviors a little."
Carol: "No, August, you minimized your behaviors a *lot*."
August: "But I think I'm ready for your program."

From the outset, this interchange illustrated policy discussions of the past several years. Most notably, August's defining himself as a "sex offender," and by implication not anything more than that label. When considering the processes by which people make difficult changes in their life, it is no surprise that many would question whether labeling others doesn't risk causing further harm. If August only thinks of himself as the sum of his worst behaviors, is it not that much more difficult for him to change? Likewise, Willis (2018) asked in an article on the ethics of labeling, in essence, "Why call them by the one thing we don't want them to be?".

Many have argued on behalf of person-first and other forms of inclusive language (American Psychological Association, 2023). In clinical applications, this can actually increase the accountability that many outsiders desire from treatment (i.e., the belief that one must acknowledge all past harms and accept the label of "sex offender" before one can change. However, it can be easy for clients to distance themselves from labels such as "offender." The logic, in the author's experience, has been along the lines of, "these people are trying to make me into something I'm not. I know I abused someone, but I'm not like those monsters I hear about. I need to push back and not accept this." At the same time, plain-English discussions about how they have harmed others may make the point more simply and directly; although in the eyes of the law they may be an offender, they are more than the sum of their offenses. Had August learned in treatment that he was someone whose actions had hurt a lot of people and that he could do the work to build a better life and possibly make amends, he might have been further ahead in treatment than on the morning that he met Emily.

August

Life had not been easy for August. His earliest years were chaotic, marked by a father who was frequently absent due to incarcerations and a mother who was dependent on alcohol and drugs. There were some indications that she had used drugs during her pregnancy with August. Nonetheless, his parents had love in their hearts for him, despite their frequent negligence. Throughout his life, there have been subtle indications that his mother may have abused him sexually at some time, but this was never confirmed, and August has never acknowledged that it happened. There were, however, allegations of sexual abuse by an uncle, and the state child welfare agency did substantiate these. Although the uncle escaped criminal prosecution, he cut off all contact with his family.

August's first years in school did not go well. He was quickly diagnosed with ADHD due to impulsivity and difficulties paying attention. These difficulties were compounded by poor relationships with his teachers, who often felt that he required more care than they could give. August was referred to psychological testing, which also identified learning disabilities in the areas of language and math, anxiety, and depressive symptoms. The focus of the evaluation, however, was on presenting issues rather than a deep understanding of August. Although accurate, it lacked explanatory depth and did not entirely convey what it was like to be August. The result was a suite of ideas for managing August in the classroom, but not for giving August a sense of connection or meaning and purpose in the world. As a result, while he received important educational attention, his interpersonal skills did not necessarily improve. Over the years, he described feeling increasingly like an outcast.

August's mother eventually became clean and sober. When August was ten years old, she started a daycare program for children in infancy to five years old in her home. August would spend his afternoons and evenings upstairs, with occasional overlap when his mother was downstairs with the children. August was somewhat aware of an emerging sense of jealousy that the children were getting most of his mother's attention and affections. He first engaged in sexual behaviors with a five-year-old when he was twelve, persuading the child to keep this a secret. These behaviors continued until he was fourteen. A child told their mother, who reported the abuse to the state's child welfare agency. August was initially placed into foster care, where he misbehaved, and then into a large, inpatient residential treatment center for youths with problematic sexual behaviors.

August did not do particularly well in this setting; aside from physical aggression towards others, he frequently engaged in behaviors such as pulling fire alarms, emptying fire extinguishers at staff members, and calling emergency services only to then hang up, resulting in the police showing up at the program. He also engaged in sexual behaviors with other residents and appeared to focus on those who were (or at least looked) younger than him. He was also prolific in accessing the internet to seek out sexually explicit materials. When discussing his life, August often stated that he felt his behaviors were reasonable and justified.

No form of sanctions appeared effective; he was released near his 18th birthday to a supervised living setting. It was while in this setting that August was caught with Child Sexual Abuse Materials (CSAM), but not prosecuted. This was primarily because he was under the guardianship of his parents and living under supervision. Upon detection of the CSAM on his computer, he attempted to kill himself with an overdose of medication, and psychiatrically hospitalized. He was released to the specialized detention center where he met Emily.

While in detention, August went through a risk assessment and received DSM-5 diagnoses of Pedophilic Disorder, non-exclusive type, and Antisocial Personality Disorder. Although technically accurate, the stigmatizing nature of these labels rendered August eligible for very few treatment or employment settings. While some aspects of this reflected common sense (for example, August should not work in environments where he has unsupervised access to children), it also meant that many avenues would be closed off to him for years to come.

What Next?

Like many in the field, Emily faced a wide range of opinions and findings about what would happen next. She and the facility director agreed that August would be a good candidate for Slate Valley, which provided a very high level of supervision and structure, while still affording supervised access to community activities, all based on the premise that clients in treatment should not be unnecessarily restricted and should be able to live each day in a meaningful fashion. The admissions process was straightforward, with documentation provided, consent forms signed, and legal logistics sorted.

From here, however, there was not as much guidance as one might hope. Emily had a copy of August's risk assessment report, which (not surprisingly) addressed the various risks that he would need to work on in treatment. In many ways, this was the easiest part of it all; there may be a greater number of established assessment measures than there are proven treatment methods.

Further, to be truly evidence-based, Emily would need to rely on a wide body of research. Evidence-based practices, as defined by the American Psychological Association (APA, 2006; 2021), involves "the integration of best available research with clinical expertise in the context of patient characteristics, culture, and presences" (APA, 2006, p. 273). In August's case, this meant that there was no empirically supported treatment protocol to follow, although the principles of effective correctional rehabilitation (including those of risk, need, responsivity; Bonta & Andrews, 2017) certainly outlined much of the way forward. To begin adhering to these principles, Emily already had much of what she needed. What was left had more to do with two fundamental questions:

- How can I best understand August?
- How can I best engage him in a treatment experience where he can make the changes he needs to his life?

The following sections offer ways forward for understanding and getting started in treatment, even under difficult circumstances.

Risks/Needs

To construct an effective treatment plan, there is no substitute for an effective assessment (Yates et al., 2010). According to August's risk assessment, and the information provided above, several risk factors became apparent:

- August had an established pattern of sexual interest in children.
- He had a long history of breaking rules and problematic behaviors.
- His behavior was often highly impulsive.
- He had few skills for building and maintaining relationships with those close to him or with acquaintances.
- August was young (20 years old at the time of his placement in Slate Valley).
- He had persisted in his problem sexual behaviors over time, at different periods of his life.
- August was prone to emotional collapses and rapidly escalating negative emotions.
- He was described (and described himself) as "sexually preoccupied."
- August had difficulties with anticipating and solving problems in his daily life.
- His coping style was one of focusing on the emotions caused by stresses rather than on finding solutions.
- August experienced himself as not fitting in anywhere and experiencing profound social isolation.
- He did not have a meaningful education or employment history.

When one looks only at August's risks and needs, a dismal portrait emerges. Ward and Stewart (2003) likened treatments that only examine risk and need to a "pin-cushion model." In this way of thinking, each risk is a pin to be removed from the individual and each need requiring treatment to "address." While there was no question in Emily's mind that the list of risk and need factors above was accurate and warranted attention, it was not full guidance for treatment.

Putting Trauma-Informed Care (TIC) into Practice

TIC has gained currency in research and practice in recent years, and entire books have been written on its application (Levenson et al., 2017). A full description is therefore beyond the scope of this chapter. Suffice it to say that August's risk/need factors offered clues to the ongoing legacy of his early life adversity.

One potential way to think about TIC is to begin by looking at the client's adverse experiences, comparing these to optimal developmental experiences, and then considering how the risk factors a client presents might represent the lingering impact of developmental insults. In no way is TIC exculpatory; rather it is a way of understanding clients and adjusting treatment to accommodate their vulnerabilities as well as meet their needs.

Take these adverse experiences from August's past:

- a history of sexual abuse
- separation from family members
- a family member's incarceration
- a family member's impairment
- neglect and apparent poverty

Then consider these three over-arching areas of normative development:

- relationship capacity (e.g., secure attachments and skills for healthy relationships)
- cognitive style and implicit theories about the world (e.g., the world can be a safe place where I can make friends and have my needs met)
- self-regulation (e.g., the ability to manage the stresses and challenges of daily life

Looking at the risk factors above, one way to understand them is as barriers to these developmental tasks. For example:

- Relationship capacity (e.g., secure attachments and skills for healthy relationships). This might include or be adjacent to the risk factors of:

  Sexual interest in children.
  He had few skills for building and maintaining relationships, either with those close to him or with acquaintances.
  August was young (20 years old) and was therefore absent deeper relationships
  His problem sexual behaviors had persisted over time, at different periods of his life.
  He was described (and described himself) as "sexually preoccupied."
  August experienced himself as not fitting in anywhere and experiencing profound social isolation.

- Cognitive style and implicit theories about the world (e.g., the world can be a safe place where I can make friends and have my needs met). This might include or be adjacent to the risk factors of:

  August had difficulties with anticipating and solving problems in his daily life.
  His cognitive style and implicit theories about the world could also be implicated in any of the other risk factors (e.g., he may possess the attitude that children can consent to sex, and that this could combine with his sexual interest in children and impulsivity to create a very serious proclivity to abuse).

- Self-regulation (e.g., the ability to manage the stresses and challenges of daily life). This might include or be adjacent to the risk factors of:

  He has a long history of breaking rules and problematic behaviors.
  His behavior was frequently highly impulsive.
  August was young (and therefore more immature).
  He had persisted in his problem sexual behaviors over time, at different periods of his life despite being aware of the consequences of his actions.
  August was prone to emotional collapses and rapidly escalating negative emotions.

He was described (and described himself) as "sexually preoccupied," frequently acting on that interest.

August had difficulties with anticipating and solving problems in his daily life.

His coping style was one of focusing on the emotions caused by stresses rather than on finding solutions.

He did not have a meaningful education or employment history.

Tying these threads together, the following portrait emerges:

- At a time when others were experiencing the warmth and caring of their first loving relationships (early childhood), August experienced absence and neglect. While some children and adolescents can overcome this, August came to view the world as a dangerous place where he was unwanted and considered unworthy. He experienced considerable social isolation and likely felt that children were among the only people who would accept him or be easily persuaded by his sexual advances. As a perceived matter of survival, he learned how to blend into his environment so that he would escape the attention of those who might abuse him.
- At a time when others were learning to read, write, and do arithmetic in school, August focused on many of his cognitive resources protecting himself from abuse and steeling himself against social rejection. With so much of his cognitive energies directed at maintaining safety, he did not have the opportunity to develop adequate skills for anticipating and solving problems, and often made decisions impulsively. It is no surprise that he would eventually lag his peers. Likewise, it is not surprising that he would experience problems with attention, anxiety, and depression.
- At a time when others were learning dating skills and the components of initiating and building closer relationships, August was working to keep himself safe within the confines of a residential treatment center, in which covert sexual behaviors were far easier to accomplish than more developmentally normative relationships.

The net result was someone whose way of responding to the world had become entrenched with inappropriate behavior. Ironically, the very way of thinking that it would take to re-adapt to his circumstances was out of reach, since August had focused on immediate threats to his safety for so long. In other words, he had spent so much of his life looking outward, constantly on guard for threats, that his capacity to observe his own thoughts and actions had never entirely developed.

Ultimately, August's early life experiences interfered with his relationship, which led to self-protective attitudes and beliefs, including some that made it more likely he would abuse again. This was accompanied by problems with self-regulation and an interactive effect of the challenges in all three areas. To the outside world, August presented as the list of risk factors above, with few people seeing him as more than the sum of his harmful actions. To August, his thoughts, behaviors, and emotional responses to circumstances had developed in response to a world that seemed filled with constant threats. For reasons that might never become clear, August had not changed these ways of responding to the world, even though the circumstances of the world around him had often changed.

Where traditional treatment programs would have simply targeted the risks/criminogenic needs directly, Emily was developing a useful understanding of how August had lived up to this point. Importantly, she had a more comprehensive formulation of how he could come to understand his life, and the world around him, differently.

Good Lives Model (GLM)

Being able to understand August's risk factors in the context of a life narrative of adversity and neglect does not directly offer a structured way forward in treatment. For a therapist like Emily, it can be useful to have an over-arching practice framework within which to work. Ward et al. (2024) have defined the GLM as, "a strengths-based approach to rehabilitation in the wake of causing harm to others and one's self. It is a strength-based rehabilitation theory and practice framework … because it is responsive to clients' particular interests, abilities, and aspirations. It also directs practitioners to explicitly construct individualized intervention plans that help corrections clients acquire the means and capabilities to achieve the things that are personally meaningful to them" (p. 525).

Central to the GLM is its twin focus both on managing risks and attaining wellbeing and various aspirations and states of being that are common to all human beings. Although the terminology may fluctuate, these aspirations and states of being, known as primary human goods, are (in no fixed order):

- life (living and surviving)
- knowledge (learning and knowing)
- excellence in work and play
- excellence in agency (autonomy and self-directedness)
- inner peace
- friendship/relatedness
- community
- spirituality (including having a sense of meaning and purpose)
- happiness (states of happiness and pleasure)
- creativity (including having new experiences)

Individuals seek these goods in a variety of means, sometimes in ways that serve their long-term interests and sometimes in ways that cause harm to self or others. The importance of each good and the means by which people seek to attain them will help to determine one's implicit or explicit *good life plan.*

In considering August's apparent good life plan (which prioritized living and surviving, friendship/relatedness, and remaining autonomous over most of the others), Emily took note of how each risk factor was implicated in the goods. For example:

- Life (living and surviving): August had implicitly sought to attain this through his self-protective actions. These included his impulsivity, rule-breaking, and the belief that the world is a dangerous place in which one must meet their own needs, since no one will help. In his original environment, this calculus for living and surviving made sense. However, his approach had the effect of keeping him in environments in which living and surviving were more difficult.

- Excellence in agency (autonomy and self-directedness). August's impulsivity and rule-breaking also served to provide him a sense of independence and that he was his own person. In his original home environment, not remaining autonomous could have been an existential threat, and so he intended to maintain this autonomy through any means necessary.
- Friendship/relatedness: August had been denied the most fundamental forms of relatedness early in his life. Growing up, he lacked the skills needed to initiate and maintain relationships. Instead, he turned to inappropriate and harmful means for achieving this good through the sexual abuse of children, sex with peers who were unable to consent, and the use of CSAM and other sexually explicit materials.
- Inner peace: August had experienced few opportunities for inner peace throughout his childhood, and eventually turned to sexual behavior as a way of regulating his mood.

While Emily did not yet have the time for a more complete examination of August's good life plan, she now had four over-arching domains in mind where she might focus a treatment plan for August. By helping August find more effective ways to attain the goods of living, relatedness, autonomy, and inner peace (as well as the others in due course), she could not only assist him in leading a more satisfying life, but also better manage his risks. For August, this approach to treatment was far more appealing than past efforts aimed at having him relinquish behaviors that caused harm to others (i.e., the "pin-cushion" approach described above).

Given all the information up to this point, how can we best understand the variables at play in August's life? To summarize the main points:

- August experienced adversity in his formative years. This adversity affected him in the areas of attachment and relationships with others. He further developed a cognitive style and implicit theories about the world based on surviving the present moment more than on developing a better future.

- His responses to this adversity involved a narrative of behaviors, diminished relational capacities, attitudes, and beliefs that from the outside appeared as "risk factors."
- These risk factors, which reflected underlying dynamic process, also served as barriers to achieving the GLM's primary human goods.
- By only focusing on risks and needs, programs had explicitly focused only on abuse-related aspects of August's life, leaving him with the belief that he was little more than a "sex offender." In this way, they had not incorporated the many states of being that August had sought to achieve or attain. By limiting interventions to risk reduction, the programs had not accounted for how achieving a better life can aid the management of risks.

By helping August to understand how the things that had happened to him had limited his life up to this point, Emily was better able to help him see that he had both the opportunity and responsibility to change his behavior.

Next Steps and Motivational Interviewing

From here, Emily used the style and spirit of Motivational Interviewing to fully establish a course of treatment. At this point, August was well engaged in treatment but looked forward to further clarity about the way forward. The GLM's focus on establishing "approach goals" that one can attain or achieve rather than avoidance goals that one seeks to avoid may not suit every client. Clients sometimes enter treatment with the explicit goal of avoiding further offending.

> August: "Look, I really like all this talk about good lives and getting past my past, but my biggest goal right now isn't about anything I can achieve, it's to not offend again. I want to avoid offending."
> Emily (using reflective listening): "Above all else, you never want to cause harm to others again."
> August: "Yes."

Emily: "So that is what it all boils down to and you want skills to prevent any further harm."
August: "Yes."
Emily: "May I share a further thought?"
August (smiling): "Of course!"
Emily: "This focus on prevention and the skills you want to learn and get better at are excellent. I hope you don't mind that preventing harm is also part of these broader goals of getting better at living and surviving (by keeping you out of trouble), relationships (because preventing harm will lead to better relationships), autonomy (because you will remain free to live your life as you please), and inner peace (because you won't be in trouble), and many other goals like happiness (because you'll be more proud of your accomplishments in this area), community (because others will be comfortable with your presence), and the list goes on. For now, though, can we agree that the number one goal of treatment is to prevent offending and that our strategies are going to involve building and practicing the skills to achieve that?"
August: "I like that plan."
Emily: "Excellent. My only request is that we check in at the start and end of every session to make sure that the work we are doing is meaningful and valuable to you, and that we are producing the intended results together."

Emily then introduced measures to ensure that the work she did aligned not only with the principles of risk, need, and responsivity, but also with the therapeutic alliance. The therapeutic alliance, first defined by Bordin (1979) involves ensuring that the therapist and client understand and are in agreement with:

- the nature of their relationship and how the therapist fits into the client's life
- the goals of treatment (in August's case, this would, over time, include all of the GLM goods)
- the tasks of treatment (which involved TIC, the GLM, micro-skills such as reflective listening from Motivational Interviewing, which Emily used above and throughout treatment, and the use of feedback methods described above)

- actively tailoring treatment to the unique characteristics, values, and cultural considerations of the client

Conclusion

August went on to make excellent progress in the Slate Valley Services program, in large part because he and Emily had attended to establishing a firm foundation to the treatment he received. After roughly a year in the program, his team determined that he would benefit from a lower level of care. He eventually entered a supervised living situation in which he had his own apartment and his therapist and case manager would visit to ensure his successful transition into the community.

By initially focusing on August's history of adversity, and understanding his risks in that context, Emily was able to establish a case formulation of his risks and treatment needs. She could then use the Good Lives Model as a practice framework for addressing these needs. By using the GLM in the service of staying trauma-informed, and actively using August's feedback on how treatment sessions were and were not effective in each instance, she and August were able to keep his treatment on track. By using the reflective listening and other skills as methods she would focus on, Emily was able to prevent the pitfalls that previous programs had experienced.

References

American Psychological Association. (2006). Evidence-based practice in psychology. *American Psychologist, 61*(4), 271–285. https://doi.org/10.1037/0003-066X.61.4.271

American Psychological Association. (2021). *Professional practice guidelines for evidence-based psychological practice in health care*. https://www.apa.org/about/policy/evidence-based-psychological-practice-health-care.pdf

American Psychological Association. (2023). *Inclusive language guide* (2nd ed.). https://www.apa.org/about/apa/equity-diversity-inclusion/language-guidelines.pdf

Bonta, J., & Andrews, D. A. (2017). *The psychology of criminal conduct* (6th ed.). Routledge.

Bordin, E. S. (1979). The generalizability of the psychoanalytic concept of the working alliance. *Psychotherapy: Theory, Research and Practice, 16*(3), 252–260. https://doi.org/10.1037/h0085885

Levenson, J. S., Willis, G. M., & Prescott, D. S. (2017). *Trauma-informed care: Transforming treatment for people who sexually abuse.* Safer Society Press.

Marshall, W. L. (2005). Therapist style in sexual offender treatment: Influence on indices of change. *Sexual Abuse: Journal of Research and Treatment, 17*(2), 109–116. https://doi.org/10.1177/107906320501700202

Miller, W. R., & Rollnick, S. (2023). *Motivational interviewing: Helping people change and grow* (4th ed.). The Guilford Press, a division of Guilford Publications, Inc.

Walters, S. T., Vader, A. M., Harris, T. R., & Jouriles, E. N. (2009). Reactivity to alcohol assessment measures: An experimental test. *Addiction, 104*(8), 1305–1310. https://doi.org/10.1111/j.1360-0443.2009.02632.x

Ward, T., & Stewart, C. A. (2003). The treatment of sex offenders: Risk management and good lives. *Professional Psychology: Research and Practice, 34*(4), 353–360. https://doi.org/10.1037/0735-7028.34.4.353

Ward, T., Willis, G. M., & Prescott, D. S. (2024). The rehabilitation of corrections clients: Good lives and risk reduction. In G. M. Davies & A. R. Beech (Eds.), *Forensic psychology: Crime, justice, law, interventions* (pp. 511–531). Wiley.

Willis, G. M. (2018). Why call someone by what we don't want them to be? The ethics of labelling in forensic/correctional psychology. *Psychology, Crime and Law, 24*, 727–743. https://doi.org/10.1080/1068316X.2017.1421640

Yates, P. M., Prescott, D. S., & Ward, T. (2010). *Applying the good lives and self regulation models to sex offender treatment: A practical guide for clinicians.* Safer Society Press.

10

Developing an EpiCrim Approach to the Prevention, Treatment and Reintegration of People Convicted of a Sexual Offence

Emily Jones and Geraldine Akerman

Introduction

The undeniable connection and prevalence of experiences of trauma leading to enduring adverse mental health consequences (and in some cases criminal behaviour), offer a strong foundation of evidence for inpatient mental health services and the prison systems to adopt a trauma-informed approach to treatment. In this chapter, the authors examine what 'trauma-informed care' (TIC) looks like within a workforce, the role it has in treatment and the documented benefits of implementation. Further, the barriers and challenges faced in creating a trauma-informed environment are discussed. One author contributes insights from their work in a prison setting, while the other draws from

E. Jones (✉) · G. Akerman
HMP Grendon, Edgcott, England
e-mail: Emily.Jones@Oxfordhealth.nhs.uk

G. Akerman
Integrated Mental Health Team, HMP Grendon, Aylesbury, UK

K. McCartan et al. (eds.), *Developing and Implementing a Public Health and Criminological Approach to Tackling Sexual Abuse*, Palgrave Studies in Risk, Crime and Society, https://doi.org/10.1007/978-3-031-93634-0_10

their experience in a hospital environment. Due to these diverse backgrounds, the terminology referring to individuals under our care or treatment is used interchangeably throughout the chapter with terms such as patient, prisoner and resident being employed based on the context.

What is Trauma-Informed Care/ Trauma-Informed Workforce?

Trauma-informed care can encompass various interpretations, and our experiences suggest that its meaning can vary among staff disciplines, clients and services. Watson et al. (2014) conceptualise trauma-informed care as that which is aware of the prevalence and adverse effects of trauma, and of the potential of retraumatising clients with trauma histories through coercive practices. A similar definition is offered by Sweeney et al. (2018) who stated that trauma-informed approaches are based on recognition and comprehensive understanding of the widespread prevalence and effects of trauma. They posit that this leads to a fundamental paradigm shift from thinking 'what is wrong with you?' to considering 'what happened to you?'. In their definition of trauma-informed care, Sweeney et al. (2018) emphasise that it transcends being merely a specific service or a set of rules. Instead, it represents a journey of organisational transformation aimed at fostering environments and relationships conducive to recovery and the prevention of retraumatisation. Lomani and Brooker (2022) developed a list of trauma-informed principles. These include not retraumatising, collaboration and mutuality, understanding the inherent power imbalance between staff and survivors, and ensure that relationships are based on mutuality, respect, trust, connection and hope. These are critical because abuse of power is typically at the heart of trauma experiences. Abuse of power often leads to feelings of disconnection and hopelessness, and because it is through relationships that healing can occur, staffs need to be sufficiently trained and supported through supervision to develop. However, despite this clarity, understanding what it looks like in practice remains a challenge. While definitions are valuable, it is equally essential to envision how it manifests and is applied in real-world scenarios.

Some researchers have outlined the features of what trauma-informed care would resemble in practical terms. The Substance Abuse and Mental Health Services Administration (SAMHSA, 2014) list the main features as an appreciation of the impact of trauma, the recognition of signs and symptoms of trauma in clients and staff, a full integration of knowledge about trauma into policies procedures and practices and a commitment to avoid retraumatisation. In a review of the literature, Muskett (2014) found and documented key principles in trauma-informed care. They are as follows (i) clients need to feel connected, valued, informed and hopeful of recovery, (ii) the connections between childhood trauma and adult psychopathology is known and understood by all staff: and (iii) staff work in mindful and empowering ways with individuals, family and friends and other social service agencies to promote and protect the autonomy of the individual. In the next section of this chapter, we explore the forensic setting as a place of work and the impact this can have on being trauma-informed. This leads us into discussing the available research into trauma-informed workforces in forensic settings and discusses its implications.

The Forensic Setting Environment

Prisons throughout the world are suffering for a range of reasons, for instance, overcrowding, lack of staff, poor working environment and decreased funding (Fair & Walmsley, 2021). While there may not be direct research drawing explicit parallels, the underlying dynamics between prisons and forensic hospitals resonate. Hospitals, like prisons, grapple with overcrowding, strained resources, inadequate staffing and funding shortages. Therefore, it is paramount that staffs are supported to do what can be very challenging work. So called 'enchanted workplaces' are those where workers feel connected to their work and are active agents in making a difference (Michaelson et al., 2014). Disenchantment can have a negative impact on the individual and organisation. This could include feelings of inequity, which may lead to increased absenteeism and attrition (Smith, 2023) which impacts on the prison regime and interventions within it. This may also impact on the relationships, connections and interactions that staffs have with those that they are caring for. In such contexts, these workplace stressors can compound the toll of working with patients who are experiencing trauma. Professionals may find themselves repeatedly exposed to emotionally charged situations which can lead to burnout, vicarious trauma and compassion fatigue.

Bierie, (2012) considered the physical prison environment and how it impacted on staff. Unpleasant physical conditions (presence of insects, rodents, dirt, litter, clutter, noise and lack of sanitation supplies) corresponded to significant problems for staff. They found staff who worked in harsher prison conditions were significantly more likely to drink and smoke, were more worried about aspects of their life outside prison, and they displayed more psychological and physical health problems. They also reported using more sick leave. Steiner and Wooldredge (2017) found that prisons which provided better conditions had far fewer reported staff problems than prisons with poorer conditions. There are also greater violence and assaults against staff in linear style prisons, (also known as "corridor prisons" where prison cells are arranged along long straight corridors) and staff working in these prisons generally perceive themselves to be working in unsafe conditions.

Mann et al. (2019) described the *rehabilitative culture* as a relational model for those in prison. This highlights the importance of procedural justice, the role of leadership, the nature of the physical environment, the value of peer mentoring, and the way in which security procedures are undertaken. Mann et al., consider how imprisonment itself cannot reduce re-offending and so the quality of the environment is paramount. By its nature, a prison can be an anti-social environment and so interventions such as a Therapeutic Community (TC), Psychologically Informed Planned Environment (PIPE), Rehabilitative Culture and Offender Personality Disorder Pathway (OPD) models seek to create such a pro-social culture. Suggestions for an effective therapeutic culture include trauma-informed interventions and having a whole-prison culture, as advised by the Trauma-informed approach (Levenson et al. 2017) alongside a culture in which staffs support the rehabilitative ethos.

How and Why Does a Trauma-Informed Approach Work?

Being trauma-informed greatly benefits compassion in treatment and treatment itself by fostering a deeper understanding and empathy for the experiences of those receiving care.[1] In this section, we discuss the ways in which being trauma-informed as a workforce develops compassion and in turn benefits treatment.

First, being trauma-informed enhances our understanding and encourages staff members to recognise that individuals' behaviour and responses may be shaped by past traumatic experiences. This understanding helps to avoid misinterpretation or judgment of patient behaviours and instead fosters empathy and compassion. Crole-Rees and et al. (2023) collected the views from staff asking what they considered to be important in a trauma-informed pathway in prison. They found three super-ordinate themes, asking what happened and how to respond, providing specialist approaches and a compassionate relational approach. Having an understanding of the compassion focussed approach knits well with the trauma-informed approach (Taylor & Akerman, 2022). Crole-Rees et al., found an improved relationship among staff and prisoners when staff knew what had happened to people they were working with. This in turn would help staff understand when prisoners responded in a certain way, had anniversaries of events and so forth. They also flagged the need for mental health screening of prisoners, so they had knowledge of their trauma histories. This helped them to cope with the interpersonal and intrapersonal impacts of trauma they experienced. Secondly, organisational factors, relating to the culture and leadership, resources and systems and processes. This included the impact of having a high turnover of staff, which prevented the development

---

[1] The terms prisoner, service-user or similar terms will be used throughout the chapter as the authors consider it important to not use stigmatising language, see Akerman (2018).

of support relationships. Thirdly, the staff factors were associated with skills development and training, staff well-being and support and staff attitudes. The respondents highlighted the importance of supervision and training. The training enabled them to understand the impact of trauma, and supervision helped them explore their own thoughts and feelings about the work. Supervision is shown to reduce stress levels and complaints, increase in staff morale, increase confidence and reduce burnout and emotional strain. Further, it is found to increase knowledge and awareness of potential solutions to clinical problems (Rothwell et al., 2021).

Second, having a workforce that is trauma-informed means having a workforce that prioritises patient autonomy and empowerment. This may manifest itself in a service that actively involves patients in decision-making processes, respecting their preferences and boundaries. This collaborative approach builds trust and fosters a sense of safety, which is essential for healing and recovery. On the surface forensic settings such as prisons and hospitals appear to lack opportunities for autonomy or choice. Mastrigt and Vansteenkiste (2017) argue that there is considerable variation in the number and type of choices offered to those incarcerated, if the workforces are willing to be open to finding them. The authors state that in doing so it has crucial importance for patients' psychological functioning. This is based on self-determination theory which maintains that when an individual's autonomy, competence and relatedness needs are met individual's experience greater motivation, well-being and productivity. Conversely, when these needs are thwarted individuals may experience diminished motivation and well-being (Deci & Ryan, 2012).

A treatment modality that places autonomy at the core of its model is therapeutic communities (TCs). The TC model has the importance of relationships at its core. These relationships are described as evocative rather than didactic, allowing individuals to understand themselves and their relationship with society through ongoing interactions with their peer community, rather than relying on expert knowledge about their situation. Research has found that therapeutic communities have lower rates of recidivism compared to other treatment modalities. Specifically, the one-year proven re-offending rate for 932 prisoners who completed this program was 39%, compared to 44% for a matched control group of similar prisoners when controlling for the most complex needs (Ministry of Justice, 2016).

Thirdly, by creating environments and workforces within that environment that are sensitive to trauma trigger and stressors, trauma-informed care minimises the risk of retraumatising patients during treatment. This approach ensures that healthcare settings feel safe and supportive, allowing patients to engage more fully in their care without fear of reliving past trauma. There is growing interest in research relating to taking a trauma-informed approach to working with those who have committed sexual offences. Research (Levenson et al., 2017) has shown that those who have committed sexual offences have experienced disproportionate trauma in their past and by keeping this in mind the interventions aimed at helping rehabilitate and reintegrate them into society would be improved. Early adversity can impact on the development of distorted thinking and maladaptive coping mechanisms (including violence). It has been shown to disrupt attachment and bonding, and this can continue into adulthood. Those who have offended are found to have much higher rates of adverse childhood experiences (ACEs) than the general population, and such events change the neurochemistry of the brain, leading to poorer functioning in adulthood. Ginot (2022) describes how parts of the brain, namely the amygdala and hippocampus are part of the circuit which process fear and anxiety. It is particularly sensitive to stress at a young age and can lead to hyperarousal. This in turn impacts ability to learn, develop relationships and so forth.

Mann et al. (2013) considered how prison staff can inadvertently or deliberately undermine attempts to provide rehabilitation in prison. They considered why prisoners convicted of sexual offences refused treatment and found that some prison staff undermined the value of treatment. This happened both overtly, by telling prisoners that therapy did not work, and covertly, by failing to provide a culture where men convicted of sexual offending felt safe enough to work on their convictions. Many of these individuals likely have histories of feeling unsafe and doubting their ability to be helped. By perpetuating an environment that reinforces these negative perceptions, the prison system risks exacerbating their trauma and hindering their ability to engage meaningfully in rehabilitation efforts. This not only undermines the effectiveness of therapeutic interventions but also perpetuates cycles of despair and hopelessness, further entrenching individuals in patterns of harmful behaviour. The use of power in relationships between staff and residents in prison can also impact such that those in custody are more likely to comply with rules if they feel they are treated in a fair way. These are the aspects most discussed in a TC setting, where rules being adhered to is a constant focus of meetings.

Fourth, being trauma-informed in turn emphasises resilience building strategies that support patients in coping with and overcoming adversity. In their paper on how to implement trauma-informed care to build resilience, Bartlett and Steber (2019) highlight how common it is to forget about resilience and protective factors when focussing on adverse childhood experiences and trauma. They highlight that staff are working in organisations that lack time and staff. This shortage creates a sense of urgency to quickly identify the "heart of the matter" often the problematic events affecting the patient. However, Bartlett and Steber (2019) state that the real "heart of the matter" lies in the resilience individuals display and how they survived their trauma. Understanding the factors that contribute to this resilience is crucial, and thus it is crucial that having a trauma-informed workforce means having a workforce that focusses on resilience as well as the trauma events. These factors can be leveraged to enhance treatment and rehabilitation. Research affirms the central role of resilience in trauma and substance use disorder. Higher resilience is related to lower levels of substance use, fewer alcohol problems and a delayed onset of substance abuse (Weiland et al., 2012). Researchers provide compelling evidence in support of the association between emotional capacities and resilience, and of resilience as a mediating factor among advanced emotional capacity, affect balance and well-being (Zeidner et al., 2011).

Trauma-Informed Approach in Practice; HMP Grendon

There are several prisons which have a unit within it which functions as a TC (see Akerman, 2019) for summary. HMP Grendon is a prison which functions as a set of five TCs, with decisions which affect the whole establishment being made by representatives of each TC. There is an Enhanced Assessment and Preparation Unit (EAPU), a wing for men with learning difficulties, a wing for men with sexual convictions and three wings on which men with a range of convictions are housed.[2] Staffs working in TCs adhere to the underlying values, healthy attachment, safety, respect, communication, interdependence, relationships, participation, process, balance and responsibility. Relationships are at the core of the work and so those who live and work in a TC work through all aspects of them. The TC model shares the view that to create a therapeutic environment it is vital that there is a sense of belonging, with a culture of enquiry, being open to feedback and being willing to process everyday interactions. For this to happen there needs to be a sense of safety and willingness to attach to a community rather than an individual. Through this attachment, the underlying distress can be explored, understood and new responses practiced. Respect is demonstrated through the use of language, how people are referred to, saying please and thank you, communicating information in a timely manner and keeping people updated. This may be in contrast to other prisons where there is less involvement by the residents in the overall decision-making affecting the establishment.

Built into the weekly regime of the establishment there are meetings to support staff in their work. This includes supervision, reflective practice and staff sensitivity. Each meeting serves a different function but generally gives the member of staff time to reflect on their position in the wing and staff team, how the work may be impacting on them, their decision making and so forth. In addition, as is the case in most establishments, there is access to occupational health, the prison care team

[2] At the time of writing this chapter one wing is closed for fire improvement work, so there are only two mixed wings.

and staff support agencies. As noted in Levenson et al. (2017) staff work hard to provide an emotionally corrective experience for those they work with, connecting with their stories, to promote a better future for them. However, this can lead to high levels of burnout, compassion fatigue, sickness, etc. They note that staffs who work with those convicted of sexual offences report stress, anxiety, vicarious traumatisation and intrusive images, and so need additional support so this does not cause them harm. Moulden and Firestone (2007) also highlight the importance of supervision and so it is vital to support staff to undertake this work.

What are the Barriers to Implementing a Trauma-Informed Workforce?

In this chapter, we have highlighted that the meaning and definition of a trauma-informed workforce is and has been subjective. In the following section of the chapter, we look at ways to objectively measure how trauma-informed a workforce is. However, it is first important to explore and acknowledge the systematic barriers that can prevent individual staff from fully engaging in trauma-informed relationships and treatment. Also, please see Eason, elsewhere (chapter 10) in this volume, for the impact of trauma on staff.

As stated previously (e.g. in Brierie, 2012) austerity measures, inadequate funding and resource shortages, especially staffing deficits, can contribute to a stressful and occasionally overwhelming work environment. Sweeney et al. (2016) discuss the frequent and unpredictable changes in public services coupled with top-down approaches and a regular plethora of new initiatives to implement. This can lead to confusion and exhaustion within the workforce. While researchers emphasise that these challenges predominantly occur in public services, it is worth noting that the authors of this chapter have also encountered similar issues within private services. Low morale and high staff turnover can prevent meaningful long-term change. Muskett (2014) acknowledged that within organisational culture there is confusion and perhaps apprehension regarding introducing trauma-informed principles into individual practice beyond the reduction of seclusion/segregation and restraint. Organisational cultures can fail to support or can actively conflict with trauma-informed working methods, for example a risk averse culture that encourages staff to manage service users using 'power-over' approaches such as deprivation of privileges. It is important to acknowledge the necessity of effectively managing people, particularly when working with a potentially dangerous population. However, it is crucial to explore all available approaches to management rather than defaulting to a power-based approach in the absence of alternatives. In addition, research has identified a number of barriers to enquiring about childhood abuse, including a belief that people want to be asked about their experiences by someone of the same gender or cultural background (Young, 2001).

Females-Jewkes et al. (2018) argue that that attempts to introduce trauma-sensitive services in establishments that are replete with hostile architecture, overt security paraphernalia, and dilapidated fixtures and fittings is futile. Using examples from healthcare and custodial settings, the article puts forward suggestions for prison commissioners, planners and architects which they believe will have novel implications for prison planning and penal practice in the UK and beyond. These suggestions are focussed on changing the environment and giving autonomy back to those residing in prisons to design their own personal space, e.g. colours of their room, hanging space for clothes and softer lighting.

The authors of this chapter can draw on their own experiences within team dynamics, to highlight barriers to a trauma-informed workforce. Staff members may struggle with unresolved trauma, hindering their ability to support others effectively. Furthermore, while learning about trauma, individuals may become overly focused on their own healing journey rather than assisting those they serve. This aligns with the concept of 'wounded healers' proposed by Jung (1961), where personal suffering compels individuals to help others. Research suggests that first-hand experience with adversity can deepen empathy, but it also poses risks of vicarious traumatisation and burnout without proper self-care (Newcomb et al., 2015). Additionally, staff may experience secondary trauma from working with those who have committed crimes, further impacting their well-being and the quality of care. This highlights the complex interplay between personal and professional trauma, underscoring the importance of addressing both for a resilient, efficient and trauma-informed workforce. This level of being informed includes recognising the significance of a staff member's own trauma and its potential impact on their work. We stress the importance of creating spaces, such as supervision sessions, to discuss these issues and feelings appropriately, preventing negative impacts on treatment. In professional practice, an apt analogy to underscore this point is akin to the safety instructions provided on an aircraft. As flight attendants advise passengers to secure their own oxygen masks before assisting others, the same principle highlights the necessity of therapists' self-care. Similarly, in the realm of therapeutic interventions, ensuring one's own well-being is paramount. Consequently, a lack of support can evoke fear and a sense of unsafety, rendering staff members unable to effectively contain others' trauma and potentially perpetuating a cycle of retraumatisation.

How do we Measure Trauma-Informed Care and the Extent the Workforce is Trauma-Informed?

Services have begun to ask questions such as "what does being trauma-informed actually mean?", "do I actually practice TIC as a member of staff?" and "doesn't TIC describe what I already do?" Some organisations offer a onetime training on TIC or train their staff in evidence-based trauma specific interventions such as trauma focussed cognitive behavioural therapy and report that the workforce is 'trauma-informed'. Others might revise their policies, train their staff and provide ongoing supervision but still wonder whether the actions have resulted in a culture that is legitimately trauma-informed. A way to do this is to objectively measure the attitudes within the work force. To date the only psychometrically evaluated tool to measure trauma-informed care attitudes is the 'Attitudes to Trauma-informed Care' (ARTIC) scale developed by Baker et al. (2016). The authors on this state that the ARTIC provides the first psychometrically reliable and valid tool to help stakeholders, researchers, practitioners, policy makers and consumers evaluate TIC and its outcomes. The ARTIC has the potential to fill a gap in the field by measuring one central component of TIC; the workforce's attitudes towards it. Specifically, the authors posit that the tool has can be used as a screening tool for prospective staff members to determine whether they possess attitudes that would be a good fit for the trauma-informed culture. The authors view this development as a significant advancement in the field, particularly for service providers dedicated to cultivating and nurturing a trauma-informed workforce.

Important Factors to Consider When Implementing TIC

Diversity and inclusion are crucial considerations within the context of a trauma-informed workforce, particularly in terms of cultural competence and intersectionality. For a workforce to be truly trauma-informed, it is imperative to understand and respect the cultural backgrounds, values and beliefs of the diverse populations they support. Chang et al. (2012) discuss 'cultural humility' in the healthcare sector, describing it as an approach to cultural competence that emphasises openness, self-awareness, and a commitment to lifelong learning. Additionally, understanding intersectionality is vital in addressing trauma within the workforce. Service users may experience multiple forms of oppression or discrimination based on factors such as race, ethnicity, gender identity, sexual orientation, socioeconomic status and disability. These experiences are traumatising in themselves, and it is imperative for the workforce to understand how these factors impact service users. Professionals lacking awareness of intersectionality risk inadvertently retraumatising individuals by failing to acknowledge the impact of discrimination. Creating safe spaces for discussing these experiences is essential for fostering healing and promoting resilience among those who have faced discrimination.

Diversity and inclusion was highlighted further during the COVID-19 pandemic, as those from ethnic minority groups were suffering more serious consequences of the virus right from the start of it (Moralis & Ali, 2021). This further underscored the need for trauma-informed care, exacerbating existing mental health issues and introducing new stressors. Research conducted just prior to the pandemic (Jaegers et al., 2020) described elevated levels of occupational burnout, depression and post-traumatic stress disorder (PTSD) among prison staff. Akerman and Jones (2021), along with Akerman et al. (2020), highlighted the impact on the therapeutic community, while Jones and Akerman (2021) discussed the impact on forensic psychologists. Despite being seen as keyworkers, staff in prisons and hospitals emerged from the pandemic feeling depleted, with heightened levels of burnout (Ward & Smith, 2023). This burnout correlates with making mistakes, which can be especially dangerous in a prison environment.

Supporting Staff Moving Forward

Berger and Quiros (2014) highlighted the need for supervision for those working in trauma-informed practice. They discussed how the principles and strategies of supervision can be adapted and applied to foster the professional and personal growth of practitioners and enhance their mastery of trauma-informed care. Supervision of trauma-informed care is comprised of educational, support and administrative guidance and oversight. However, the constant interaction with traumatised clients may have negative effects on practitioners and therefore some elements of trauma-informed practice supervision require special attention.

To support staff well-being, Mason and Morris (2023) found that local awards acknowledging staff value, strategic thinking about improving job satisfaction, access to training, supervision and debriefs after incidents were beneficial. By integrating principles of diversity, inclusion and lessons learned from the COVID-19 pandemic, trauma-informed care can be more effectively implemented, ensuring comprehensive and adaptable support for both service users and providers.

More recently, the Trauma Risk Management (TRiM) model was introduced to prisons and hospitals. It was developed by military personnel (Jones et al., 2003). Previously trained counsellors or debriefers had attended staff who had experienced a traumatic event soon after it occurred. However, this was not found to be useful, as the feedback was that personnel preferred to talk to people they knew, and who understood the setting they were working in. Also, after a period of time the initial response had subsided and having the debrief too soon had not been helpful. They found that organisational resilience was a result of the relationship between individuals in it, rather than factors within the individuals (Jones et al., 2012*)*. They acknowledged the need for a period of 'watchful waiting' and the offer of additional support should it be required. This process offers the individual contact with a trained colleague (a TRiM Practitioner) to assess for any signs or symptoms of distress following the incident. This takes place around a month after the incident. Having meetings with peers is seen to reduce any stigma related to seeking support. The meeting is an opportunity for the partitioner to have a structured conversation (not therapy or counselling) in a safe place, with a peer. This is followed with another meeting approximately a month later and scores of signs will be reassessed. Should further referrals be required they would be made, to for instance to Occupational Health or the service's Psychological team. This service is currently being evaluated in hospital and prison settings, but initial findings have been positive.

Conclusion

In conclusion, adopting a trauma-informed approach within both inpatient mental health services and the prison system is essential for addressing the pervasive impact of trauma on individuals. This approach requires a comprehensive understanding of trauma's prevalence and effects as well as a commitment to fostering environment that prioritise safety, respect and empowerment. Being trauma-informed is important because it enhances empathy, it improves patient-staff relationships and improves treatment outcomes. Delivering trauma-informed care can be hard and there are significant challenges such as resource constraints that limit the availability of necessary training and support, organisational resistance to change which can stem from entrenched practices and attitudes, and the complexity of integrating trauma-informed care into existing systems.

Prisons and secure hospitals can be retraumatising for staff as well as prisoners and patients. Working with people who are traumatised can have a profound impact on staff. The impact can be pernicious and develop gradually, such that the individual is not aware of it until they become burnt out or suffer compassion fatigue (see Eason's chapter). To enable trauma-informed care, it is important that staffs are supported with space and time to think about the impact they are having on those they are working with, and vice versa to stop the cycle of trauma. It is also important for them to have time to process the impact of the work and the transferred feelings, so they are not acting on them. Those who are mentally unwell can be aggressive towards those who are caring for them, and this can have an impact on staff morale. Staffs need to find a way to see past the actions and continue to care for the individual so it is vital for support to be offered.

Ultimately, creating a trauma-informed workforce is a journey of organisational and professional transformation that demands continuous learning, cultural competence and resilience building strategies and spaces. By addressing both individual, team and systemic barriers workforces can cultivate a supportive environment conducive to healing and recovery for all individuals impacted by trauma.

References

Akerman, G. (2018). 'I am not my offence': The importance of how we refer to service users. *Forensic Update, 1*(129), 5–8.

Akerman, G. (2019). Communal living as the agent of change. In D. Polaschek, A.Day & C.Hollin (Eds.). *(Chapter 37, pp590-602) The Wiley International Handbook of Correctional Psychology*. Wiley Blackwell.

Akerman, G. A., Jones, E., Talbot, H., & Grahame-Wright, G. (2020). Social distancing in a social therapy environment. *Therapeutic Communities: The International Journal of Therapeutic Communities, 41*(3/4), 113–127.

Akerman, G., & Jones, E. (2021). The impact of Covid-19 on forensic psychologists. *Forensic Update, 137.*

Baker, C. N., Brown, S. M., Wilcox, P. D., Overstreet, S., & Arora, P. (2016). Development and psychometric evaluation of the attitudes related to trauma-informed care (ARTIC) scale. *School Mental Health, 8*, 61–76.

Bierie, D. M. (2012). The impact of prison conditions on staff well-being. *International Journal of Offender Therapy and Comparative Criminology, 56*(1), 81–95.

Bartlett, J. D., & Steber, K. (2019). How to implement trauma-informed care to build resilience to childhood trauma. *Trauma, 9*(10).

Chang, E. S., Simon, M., & Dong, X. (2012). Integrating cultural humility into health care professional education and training. *Advances in Health Sciences Education, 17*(2), 269–278.

Crole-Rees, C., Tomlin, J., Kalebic, N., Collings, M., Roberts, N. P., & Forrester, A. (2023). An exploration of staff views of a trauma-informed pathway in a sentenced and remand prison. *The Journal of Forensic Practice, 25*(4), 420–436.

Deci, E. L., & Ryan, R. M. (2012). Self-determination theory. *Handbook of Theories of Social Psychology, 1*(20), 416–436.

Fair, H., & Walmsley, R. (2021). *World Prison Population List.* Institute for Crime and Justice Policy Research.

Ginot, E. (2022). *Our anxious selves: Neuropsychological processes and their enduring influence on who we are (Norton Series on Interpersonal Neurobiology).* WW Norton and Company.

Jaegers, L. A„ Ahmad, S. O., Scheetz, G., Bixler, E., Nadimpalli, S., Barnidge, E., Katz, I. M., Vaughn, M. G.,& Matthieu, M. M. (2020). Total Worker Health® Needs Assessment to Identify Workplace Mental Health Interventions in Rural and Urban Jails. *American Journal of Occupational Therapy, 74*(3), 1–12. https://doi.org/10.5014/ajot.2019.036400. PMID: 32365308; PMCID: PMC7198237.

Jones, E., & Akerman, G. (2021). The impact of Covid-19 on forensic psychologists. *Forensic Update, 1*(137), 25–28. https://doi.org/10.53841/bpsfu.2021.1.137.25

Jones, N., Roberts, P., & Greenberg, N. (2003). Peer-group risk assessment: A post-traumatic management strategy for hierarchal organizations. *Occupational Medicine, 53*, 469–475.

Jones, N., Seddon, R., Fear, N. T., McAllister, P., Wessely, S., & Greenberg, N. (2012). Leadership, cohesion, morale and the mental health of UK armed forces in Afghanistan. *Psychiatry, 75*(1), 49–59.

Jung, C. G. (1961). *Memories, dreams and reflections.* Fontana.

Levenson, J. S., Willis, G. M., & Prescott, D. S. (2017). *Trauma-informed care. Transforming treatment for people who have sexually abused.* Safer Society Press. ISBN 978-194023408-3.

Mason, R., & Morris, L. (2023). Health and wellbeing of healthcare staff in prisons: Joining practice reflections and the academic literature. *Prison Service Journal, 268*, 45–51.

Mann, R., Barnett, G., Box, G., Howard, F. F., O'Mara, O., Travers, R., & Wakeling, H. (2019). Rehabilitative culture in prisons for people convicted of sexual offending. In *Sexual Crime and the Experience of Imprisonment* (pp. 1–33).

Mann, R. E., Webster, S. D., Wakeling, H. C., & Keylock, H. (2013). Why do sex offenders refuse treatment? *Journal of Sexual Aggression, 19*(2), 191–206.

Michaelson, C., Pratt, M., Grant, A., & Dunn, C. (2014). Meaningful work: Connecting business ethics and organization studies. *Journal of Business Ethics, 121*, 77–90.

Ministry of Justice. (2016). Justice Data Lab Re-offending analysis: Phoenix Futures- Therapeutic Communities Programme. Open Government Licence. https://assets.publishing.service.gov.uk/media/5a80d49040f0b62302695bd6/phoenix-futures-report.pdf

Moralis, D. R., & Ali, S. N. (2021). COVID-19 and disparities affecting ethnic minorities. *The Lancet, 397*(10286), 1684–1685. https://doi.org/10.1016/S0140-6736(21)00949-1. Epub 2021 Apr 30. PMID: 33939952; PMCID: PMC9755653.

Muskett, C. (2014). Trauma-informed care in inpatient mental health settings: A review of the literature. *International Journal of Mental Health Nursing, 23*(1), 51–59. https://doi.org/10.1111/inm.12012

Newcomb, M., Burton, J., Edwards, N., & Hazelwood, Z. (2015). How Jung's concept of the wounded healer can guide learning and teaching in social work and human services. *Advances in Social Work and Welfare Education, 17*(2), 55–69.

Rothwell, C., Kehoe, A., Farook, S. F., & Illing, J. (2021). Enablers and barriers to effective clinical supervision in the workplace: A rapid evidence review. *British Medical Journal Open, 11*(9), Article e052929.

Smith, L. (2023). Losing faith in the service: A path to disenchantment among governor Grades. *Prison Service Journal, 268*, 11–16.

Steiner, B., & Wooldredge, J. (2017). Individual and environmental influences on prison officer safety. *Justice Quarterly, 34*, 324–349.

Substance Abuse and Mental Health Service Administration (SAMSHA) Trauma and Justice Strategic Initiative. (2014). *SAMHSA's concept of trauma and guidance for a trauma-informed approach.* HHS Publication No. SMA, 14-4384.

Sweeny, A., Clement, S., & Filson, B. (2016). Trauma-informed mental health-care in the UK, what is and how can we further its development. *Mental Health Review Journal, 21*, 174–192.

Sweeney, A., Filson, B., Kennedy, A., Collinson, L., & Gillard, S. (2018). A paradigm shift: Relationships in trauma-informed mental health services. *British Journal of Psychiatric Advances, 24*(5), 319–333. https://doi.org/10.1192/bja.2018.29

Taylor, J., & Akerman, G. (2022). Compassion focused cultures: Introducing compassion into a democratic therapeutic community. *Abuse: An International Impact Journal, 3*(2), 24–45.

Ward, S., & Smith, L. (2023). Burnout among prison officers: The relationship between PTSD, depression and resilience. *Prison Service Journal, 268*, 23–30.

Watson, S., Thorburn, K., Everett, M., Fisher, K., & R. (2014). Care without coercion-mental health rights, personal recovery and trauma-informed care. *Australian Journal of Social Issues, 49*, 529–549.

Weiland, B. J., Nigg, J. T., Welsh, R. C., Yau, W-Y. W., Zubieta, J-K., Zucker, R. A., & Heitzeg, M. M. (2012). Resiliency in adolescents at high risk for substance abuse: Flexible adaptation via subthalamic nucleus and linkage to drinking and drug use in early adulthood. *Alcoholism: Clinical and Experimental Research, 36*(8), 1355–1364. https://doi.org/10.1111/j.1530-0277.2012.01741.x

Young, M., Read, J., & Barker-Collo, S. (2001). Evaluating and overcoming barriers to talking about abuse histories. *Professional Psychology. Research and Practice, 32*, 407–414.

Zeidner, M., Matthews, G., & Roberts, R. D. (2011). The emotional intelligence, health, and well-being nexus: What have we learned and what have we missed? *Applied Psychology Health and Wellbeing, 4*(1), 1–30. https://doi.org/10.1111/j.1758-0854.2011.01062.x

11

Keeping Practitioners Safe: Looking After the Health and Wellbeing of the Criminal Justice Professional and Compassion Fatigue

Anne Eason

Introduction

Practitioners who work with those who have committed crimes are inevitably exposed to traumatic events or accounts of traumatic criminality. This is not just confined to healthcare professionals but extends to those frontline officers of the criminal justice sector, whose role it is to protect the public and prevent and/or reduce further crime or harmful behaviour. Sexual abuse and sexual violence are recognised as a crime type that can cause significant trauma to direct victims but also vicarious trauma those who work with them (Ogińska-Bulik & Juczyński, 2021; Ricciardelli et al., 2023; Maguire & Sondhi, 2024) in often 'unpredictable environments' (Harrison & Nichols, 2023, p. 4).

Individual trauma is defined by the Substance Abuse and Mental Health Services (SAMHSA) as the result of:

A. Eason (✉)
University of the West of England, Bristol, England
e-mail: anne.eason@uwe.ac.uk

K. McCartan et al. (eds.), *Developing and Implementing a Public Health and Criminological Approach to Tackling Sexual Abuse*, Palgrave Studies in Risk, Crime and Society, https://doi.org/10.1007/978-3-031-93634-0_11

> an event, series of events, or set of circumstances that is experienced by an individual as physically or emotionally harmful or life threatening and that has lasting adverse effects of the individual's functioning and mental, physical, social, emotional, or spiritual wellbeing.
>
> (SAMHSA, 2014, p.7)

It is experienced as uniquely as the individual and the event itself (MIND, 2023). It can be caused naturally, such as a weather disaster or epidemic or by people, accidentally or intentionally (SAMHSA, 2014). Acute trauma is associated with a one-off event whereas complex trauma refers to the repeated trauma that can be observed in victims of, for example, sexual or domestic violence or abuse. This is particularly so within the family context and adverse childhood experience (ACEs) where vulnerability, proximity and access facilitate opportunities for repeat victimisation (though other settings should not be excluded). Common responses to trauma have been observed as a broad set of emotions such as fear or shame, anger or anxiety and can be experienced at both ends of the spectrum; being overwhelmed with emotion or a numbness with little or no feelings, or detachment from any associated thoughts or memories of the event (Graham-Kevan et al., 2015). It can also manifest into different types of behaviour including avoidance, flashbacks or nightmares, mood swings or a change in thinking and attitudes, all of which can result in mental health issues such as PTSD (Post-Traumatic Stress Disorder) and have a damaging impact on everyday life.

Those working with *victims* of trauma have been the focus of research and staff interventions (Frost & Scott, 2022) due to the obvious link to exposure within the therapeutic and support environment. Nonetheless, frontline criminal justice professionals such as police, probation and prison officers are also continually exposed to traumatic events through their interactions with offenders. This can be as direct trauma (as a victim of an assault, witnessing an assault or violent aftermath), or indirectly, as secondary, or vicarious trauma (listening to a recount of a sexual or sexually violent offence, reading of a report or victim-impact statement, exposure to child-pornographic images, delivery of accredited programmes for sexual and violent offending, etc.,) (Rhineberger-Dunn et al. 2016). As such, they, too, are vulnerable to experiencing similar symptoms from direct trauma but also those associated with secondary or vicarious trauma, those that are often associated with compassion fatigue (Foley & Massey, 2021; Hilinski-Rosick et al., 2023). Drawing from a mixed vantage point of the authors own experience of trauma, previous experience as a senior probation officer and current role as a leader in police education, this chapter explores how there has been a shift in agency practices to integrate a trauma-informed philosophy that is aligned with the six principles as outlined by SAMHSA (2014). This shift recognises staff vulnerability to compassion fatigue that can support individual recovery but can also influence organisational culture change, bringing to life some of the real challenges faced by police, probation and prison officers.

Health and Well-Being

The health and wellbeing of police officers is often reported on by organisations such as Oscar Kilo (OK) and the Police Federation England and Wales (PFEW), who highlight the difficulties and impact of 'the job' on individuals and the organisation more generally. Evidence suggests "that police officers are at a high risk of mental and physical strain" (Clements et al., 2021, p. 82) and Phythian et al. (2022) identify the prevalence in serving officers is potentially far greater than is being reported, subsequently raising concerns regarding the consistency of support offered to them. With figures of between 400 and 600 traumatic incidents being attended by an individual officer across their career, a staggering 100 times more than the average adult across their lifetime (Avon & Somerset Police Federation, 2021), the health impact is inevitably significant. The headline findings from the PFEW Demand, Capacity and Welfare Survey (2020) show a range of issues faced in contemporary policing practices including understaffing, cancellation of rest days and holiday, and continuous fatigue. Coupled with the stressors of attending traumatic incidents such as death by murder, natural causes, suicide, performing death notifications, rape and other sexual assault scenes and victims, the demands made on officers substantially limit their capacity to recover or take stock of their own wellbeing and have led to growing numbers of long-term sickness (Phythian et al., 2022).

Amongst the prison and probation services, reports suggest that most are operating at least 100% above capacity (Symonds, 2023); "workloads and long hours remain pertinent issues" (Phillips et al., 2020, p. 9) and continue to be problematic as evidenced in a recent HMIP (2024) report that highlights caseloads 123.8% higher than the regional average across one South Eastern area and staffing levels at 90%. In an interview with Smith (2023) Chris Jennings, Executive Director Wales for HMP Prison and Probation Services (HMPPS) and Chair of the HMPPS Wellbeing group described the health and wellbeing of prison staff as challenging both physically and mentally, particularly when continually working with some of the most dangerous people in society. Clements and Kinman (2023, p. 18) report high incidences of sexual harassment, sexual and physical assault, and other types of traumatising behaviour targeted on prison workers that were connected to "emotional exhaustion, poorer quality sleep and work-life conflict". Therefore, rather like their police colleagues, prison and probation officers are also frequently exposed to traumatic incidents that have a longer-lasting effect, alongside the emotional lethargy associated with compassion fatigue.

Compassion Fatigue

The term compassion fatigue is "used interchangeably with burnout, vicarious traumatization, traumatic countertransference, and secondary traumatic stress" (Rhineberger-Dunn et al., 2016, p. 640) and is increasingly acknowledged amongst frontline criminal justice professionals (Grant et al., 2019; Lewis et al., 2013; Frost & Scott, 2022). In Frost and Scott's recent review of 11 research articles that explored compassion fatigue amongst criminal justice practitioners, they found that all studies identified it within those who worked directly with offenders, regardless of role or setting. By the very nature of criminal justice work, police, probation and prison personnel are regularly exposed to traumatic events or involved in incidents that are highly stressful and require "instantaneous life or death decisions" (Violanti et al., 2017, p. 643). They are also governed by a legislative and policy framework that is often restrictive, contrary to the purpose of the organisation and target driven by key performance indicators (KPIs) that are linked to political objectives and cash incentives. However, they are also subjected to the impact of increased crime rates and criminal justice crises, such as prison overcrowding. These can cause additional pressures, asking practitioners to work against the ethos or purpose of their role.

The impact of such crises or directives is substantial. For example, the directive from the National Police Chiefs Council (NPCC), instructing police officers to not make any 'non-priority' arrests (Miller et al., 2021). 'Non-priority' is defined by the NPCC as those that do not pose a high risk of reoffending or serious harm, and also planned operations. Of course on the ground, non-priority is at the discretion of the officer (or their team Sergeant) but how is that decided? Criminal damage might be considered a non-priority crime, but to the victim, it may form a pattern of sustained anti-social behaviour aimed to intimidate or harass. An arrest for them may be a high priority. Whilst the officer may recognise this and want to take appropriate action, the directive suggests it does not meet the criteria of 'priority'. Likewise, the Early Release scheme (Beard, 2023) releasing some prisoners before the automatic release point or plan 'Early Dawn' (Ministry of Justice, HMPPS and Lord Timpson, 2024) to delay court hearings to ensure prison availability, also have a direct impact. Both put inordinate strain on an already struggling police and probation service who jointly manage offenders in the community, increasing anxiety and already overwhelming caseloads, leading to compassion fatigue.

In police officers, compassion fatigue is also a potential by-product of work-related trauma. Burnett et al. (2020, p. 384) describe this as where the demand for compassion is profuse and beyond an "individual's capacity" but also a reaction to indirect exposure to trauma as part of their everyday duties (Orginska-Bulik & Juczynski, 2021). The impact of this trauma has shown to have resulted in high levels of compassion fatigue within British police officers that can lead to physical and emotional exhaustion, feelings of hopelessness, cynicism and negatively impacting on decision-making and other vital competences required to police effectively. They go on to suggest that the workflow patterns in police forces may also have an impact, worsening certain aspects through sleep deprivation and a lack of external social contact or opportunities to decompress. The University of Cambridge (2024), report that more than 90% of police officers in the UK have reportedly experienced traumatic incidents, many of whom (20%) have long-term mental health issues such as PTSD, as a direct result. However, disclosure of sexual abuse and sexual violence, particularly regarding child sexual abuse can prove very demanding, requiring the ability to detach emotionally from the evidence and accounts when investigating and processing such incidents. For police officers, exposure is often repeated sometime after, when they are required to give evidence in court, arguably re-traumatising them through the recounting of the investigation process, interviewing the suspect, gathering and evaluating the evidence, working with the victim(s) and the inevitable cross-examination of their findings.

Probation and prison officers have a different type of working relationship with sexual offenders. Much like those professionals in healthcare, the criminal justice supervisory relationship often involves repeated disclosure of detailed accounts of sexual deviance and sexual violence that the probation officer, whether working in custody or the community, will need to listen to. This may be within an accredited programme scenario or a one-to-one supervision session. Furthermore, in preparing risk assessments such as OASys Sexual reoffending Predictor (OSP) (HMPPS, 2020) and reports such as pre-sentence or parole reports, the details of the offence provide an integral element, not only exposing the officer to detailed content, but having to critically analyse it within the framework of risk management and public protection. This repetitive exposure can lead to compassion fatigue, gradually wearing down the internal resilience of the practitioner. This is reinforced by Lewis et al. (2013) who highlight how probation officers who work with violent and sexual offenders are more likely to suffer with compassion fatigue than those who work with other types of offenders.

The professionalism of the probation role demands a non-judgemental approach that assists the offender to unpick their offence, identify criminogenic triggers, and explore ways in which they can be managed or overcome (Canton, 2011). Empowering desistance is the central tenet, the principle that feeds into the reduction of harm. The EpiCrim approach supports the probation officer through the provision of health interventions that can facilitate the offender's journey in tackling issues such as substance misuse and mental health, both of which feature significantly as criminogenic factors to sexually harmful behaviours. However, an added dimension to the probation officer's exposure to trauma is where the offender themselves has suffered abuse. This subsequently becomes one of those criminogenic needs leading to further disclosure and for which there is little or no specialist intervention available (Senker, Eason and McCartan, *inpress*). For this latter issue the probation officer not only has to disregard any self-emotions about the offender's index offence but then empathise with them if they are to effectively support them in the recovery of their own sexual trauma. This can be termed as *emotional labour* where the professional must "supress some emotions and emphasise others" (Phillips et al., 2020, p. 5). Indeed, to maintain professional boundaries when working with this group can require the regular suppression of particularly negative emotions, to ensure a non-judgemental and balanced approach that breeds trust and positive change. Multiply this by high volume caseloads (Page & Robertson, 2022) and high-level accountability, and compassion fatigue is inevitable.

Similarly, prison officers work closely with the prison population and in certain vulnerable person (VP) wings and specific prisons, such as HMP Whatton, predominantly sexual offenders. Their relationship with these men is required to be positive and inclusive, creating an environment that is "pro-social, engaged and rehabilitative" (McCartan, 2022, p. 10.), facilitative of the interventions required to meet the criminogenic needs of the individual. As with probation officers, they still encounter disclosure, must be fully briefed on offending behaviour (read case files) whilst managing the often-difficult dynamics of the prison environment. This coupled with the high level of physical attacks on officers as reported by Clements and Kinman (2023), the likelihood of compassion fatigue is significant. With both prison and probation officers, however, the added dimension of their work is the extent of intensive time they have to spend with an individual, according to length of sentence. This can be from months to sometimes years working with them on their offences but also on any personal trauma they may have experienced, resulting in a conflict of emotions having to provide support despite the serious harm they have caused (Phillips et al., 2020).

The strain of conflicting emotions can prove complex and problematic to unravel because as Uzieblo (2024) points out, for many professionals, discussing their work with sexual offenders can be uncomfortable and challenging because it is misunderstood, not only by the public (Harper et al., 2022) but also by colleagues. The act of conversational debrief therefore, can often be stunted or confined to a select few who themselves may be suffering with compassion fatigue. This process has been further curtailed in the police context where police bars have closed, removing the informal setting for that conversational debrief and peer support—an environment within which they were previously able to 'let go' of some of those symptomatic emotions and strengthen personal and collective resilience. Evidently, there are practitioners in all roles that appear more resistant to compassion fatigue, this could be through what Burnett et al. (2020, p. 385) call "mental toughness" or "compassion satisfaction"; the ability to only absorb and respond to the positive feeling of reward to helping people. In the case of the probation or prison officer, this could simply relate to a sexual offender refining self-management mechanisms that reduce the likelihood of further harmful behaviour. For the police officer, the use of a risk order and seeing the behavioural change away from harmful associations. But even sharing these achievements can be problematic. For those with mental toughness, the vulnerability of their colleagues may not be recognised and so such discussions might intensify symptoms rather than release them.

The likelihood and prevalence of compassion fatigue is therefore difficult to manage and/or measure. It can have a detrimental effect on the health and wellbeing of our frontline practitioners whilst also impacting on the effectiveness of the essential work they do to protect the public, find justice for victims and promote the recovery of sexual offenders in both their own health and their ability to desist.

How is Compassion Fatigued Identified or Recognised by Staff

One of the obstacles to identifying compassion fatigue is the varied responses of the individual to trauma exposure. To help with this in policing, the University of Cambridge have created a Police Trauma Exposure Checklist (PTEC) (Miller et al. 2021, p. 217) which "provides a new UK-relevant, up-to-date list of the most frequent 'worst' experiences reported" by both police officers and police staff. The checklist can help identity those officers most at risk of trauma impact such as compassion fatigue through a hierarchical ranking of exposures, categorised as either a "traumatic event" or "situational context" (p. 216). Traumatic events are listed 1–10 from those involving children including child death, abuse and/or sexual exploitation to vicarious trauma through exposure to illicit imagery, or toxic substances (including Covid-19). Those aligned to situational context extend across a slightly shorter range from attending a "gruesome" scene involving dismembered bodies or other types of injury to working with victims who are depraved or involve vulnerable groups such as the elderly or animals. As we can see the breadth of traumatic incident attended by police is vast and this list is by no means exhaustive but built upon the responses of 1531 UK officers, and illustrates the most frequently reported 'worst' traumatic exposure. The matrix can be used to inform future workload, general wellbeing assessments and inhouse interventions such as Trauma Risk Management (TRiM) that may lead to further diagnostic assessments that can confirm and support the officer.

Of course, exposure to traumatic incidents, whether an event or the aftermath is an accepted "occupational hazard" (Foley & Massey, 2021, p. 299) by most officers and is, essentially, expected due to the nature of the role. However, the impact has been less anticipated or at least lacked focus, until more recently. As such, incidences are not recorded systematically, especially in relation to vicarious trauma and thus the true extent of those who may be affected and/or suffering with compassion fatigue is unclear. Moreover, cultural issues may be an obstacle for many individuals who may not recognise or want to acknowledge feelings associated with it.

The work of Turner (2023) gives a contemporary explanation of police culture as a collective set of beliefs, that frame police working practices through which they share an understanding of the unpredictability of policing and experiences. This explanation sits well within the idea of individual and collective ideas of identity which Papazoglou and Tuttle (2018) suggest is set within a framework of masculinity, based on a set of subcultural values and beliefs of individual strength and sense of duty to protect the 'weaker' public. However, this intense and arguably untenable mindset is, they suggest, the greatest challenge to their ability and willingness to admit to or seek help for any psychological trauma. Admission of compassion fatigue would be perceived as weak, contrary to their cultural unity or professional solidarity, viewing the health professionals there to support them as "adversaries rather than allies" (p. 3).

In prison and probation settings, compassion fatigue can be identified in the high turnover of staff sickness and employment rates (Page & Robertson, 2022). The Ministry of Justice (2019) report 34.7% of absences across HMPPS in the year to 30 September 2019 were due to mental and behavioural disorders with probation officers losing 50.2% of working days. The overall resignation rate for the same period was 6.4%. In their systematic review of literature around work-related distress in those working in correctional settings, Page and Robertson (2022) concluded that its prevalence in the workforce suggests that working with the offending community impacts on the well-being of the officers. Whilst this does not focus specifically on those who work sexual offenders, it is indicative of the stressors of working in the custodial and rehabilitative environment and how, although predictive factors such as gender, ethnicity and age could be associated with levels of different symptoms of compassion fatigue, as with policing they are a by-product of the demand for compassion and empathy exacerbated by high workloads and the need for clinical intervention.

Influences on Compassion Fatigue

Whilst elements of the criminal justice practitioner role have already been identified as influential to compassion fatigue—reading and re-reading of files, multiple exposure to pornographic imaging, sustained and long-term working relationships with violent and sexually violent offenders exploring their own traumatic experiences, and of course, physical and sexual assault—there are other more subtle influences (see Fig. 11.1).

Personal Trauma

It is with interest that Page and Robertson (2022) found that none of the research papers reviewed, considered the impact of officer's personal trauma on their overall susceptibility to compassion fatigue. Personal trauma such as a family bereavement, divorce, crime victimisation, can be highly influential to its onset in any individual. Having to navigate symptoms of one's own trauma whilst working in the volatile environment of

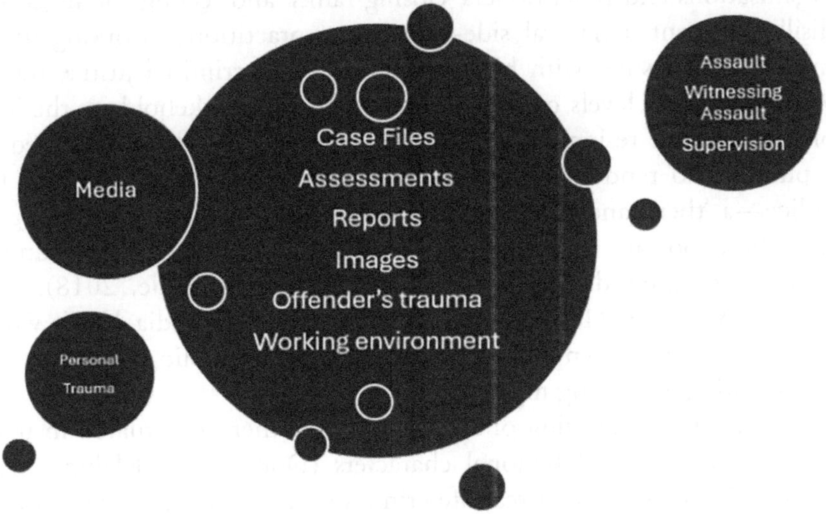

Fig. 11.1 Influences on compassion fatigue

the criminal justice system with offenders who are also traumatised, is especially difficult. Compassion fatigue increases emotionality, hindering decision-making and cognitive negativity. These could have a negative impact on prison and probation officers' effectiveness to manage situations and tasks such as risk assessment, which are vital to the successful supervision of high risk of harm offenders whether in the community or in custody. Similarly, it could impact on the police officer's ability to work effectively in their role of law enforcement (College of Policing, 2018). Trauma experienced by the practitioner must be considered in any diagnosis of compassion fatigue and performance capability.

Media

The role of the media cannot be understated both in relation to cultural solidarity and individual self-determination. Media portrayals of police, probation and prison officers, the establishments and their performance, is undisputably critical. The blame culture of British media is fuelled by political and public scrutiny and its burden, a heavy weight, individually and organisationally (Jewkes, 2011). This inevitably leads to organisations and practitioners 'closing ranks' and feelings of anger and disillusionment a natural side-effect; as a practitioner working under inordinate pressure, with high workloads, rigid criminal justice frameworks and high levels of disparagement from all stakeholders, the level of sickness and resignation is unsurprising. This is all underpinned by a public who tend to have divisive attitudes, particularly towards the police—a 'them and us' mentality—not recognising or acknowledging that they, too, are members of the community and with little understanding of their day-to-day role (Papazoglou & Tuttle, 2018). This is what Manning (1997, p. 26) referred to as a 'media loop', where police action is shown out of context, distorting public perception and perpetuating a policing mythology.

This misunderstanding of roles is often further perpetuated in inappropriately portrayed fictional characters (Donovan & Klahm, 2015; Jewkes, 2011) and using real-life crime for entertainment programmes. Kohm (2009) framed the latter as 'infotainment', playing to the sense of public justice but also the symbolic misconceptions of what these practitioners *actually* do. This can be seen in the News of the World naming and shaming campaign which peaked in 2000 following the abduction and murder of Sarah Payne and which vilified the use of Approved Premises for the housing and management of child sex offenders. This was disastrous to the safe supervision of very high-risk offenders in the community (Jewkes, 2011). More importantly, however, it put probation under the spotlight and created an environment of high alert and anxiety; fielding media phone calls, photographers and heightened emotions of residents placed additional stress on those establishments that were able to continue operating. The backlash was greater numbers of child sex offenders being housed in those Approved Premises that were not targeted, increasing already high caseloads and probation officers bearing the brunt of the paedophile 'moral panic'.

These episodes of media intensity arguably play a pivotal role in compassion fatigue. Criminal justice is vocational work, like nursing or paramedic; for the desire to help people, make a difference, serve the community and thus great pride is taken in the way in which practitioners conduct their work. The scrutiny imposed on police officers is perhaps more frequent and quite different than the others, often skewed for sensationalisation and bystander social media narratives (Ellis, 2021), narratives that are often part of a wider complaint or agenda. This is what Ellis refers to as "sousveillance of public order policing—the watching from below [...] a potent manifestation of policing's new visibility" (p. 163). Such national and intense media critique, which is frequently ill-informed as to the role of the practitioner and service within which they work, merely feeds the public with misleading information, inflating a blame culture that damages practitioners, and the trust of the public.

Trauma-Informed Organisations

For an organisation to be 'trauma-informed' it needs to have incorporated the six SAMHSA (2014) principles of safety, trust and transparency, a culture of peer support and collaboration, empowerment, voice and choice and inclusive of cultural, historical and gender issues

(Senker et al., 2023). The SAMHSA approach strives "to resist re-traumatization of clients as well as staff" (p. 10) promoting organisational practices that are considerate of the lived experience of both client and practitioner. To form such an organisational culture, therefore, not only do the signs of compassion fatigue need to be understood, but an environment that encourages safety and empowerment in vulnerability, listening to those individuals and the difficulties they are experiencing and providing appropriate services that can support them (Bristol North Somerset and South Gloucestershire, 2021). The organisation would need to have the resources and skills to manage workloads that consider individual difference, cultural and religious idiosyncrasies and gender specific issues.

Efforts have been made across the sector to raise awareness of trauma symptoms and how we can work more effectively to support those affected by it but these challenges and solutions are complex. Clements et al's. (2021) report attempts to gain an insight into the challenges faced by officers but this has proven difficult for individual forces, due to poor response rates. Furthermore, in their own research, there was conflicting evidence and interrelated issues between workload, poor management and reduced workforce numbers. There was some positivity about culture change around the safety of disclosure, but there were still fears expressed around negative repercussions and stigma. In the work of Memon et al. (2023) who looked at the well-being of prison staff, they found "concerning levels" of compassion fatigue particularly during the Covid-19 pandemic where practitioners were responsible for the imposition of more severe restrictive measures of the prison population. The stress of infection, passing on infection and the continued exposure to work-related trauma and high workload resulted in increased levels of reported compassion fatigue but little organisational support; "less than 14% of our sample reported that they had received support during the pandemic" (p. 368). This still does not appear to have been addressed (Clements & Kinman, 2023).

Conclusion

At the time of concluding this chapter, police officers in Southport were called to an incident of multiple stabbings, involving nine children and two adults, and that were committed by a child. The very next day, the same officers were called to a public order incident, instigated by the far right, around the same stabbing. Misinformation on social media had fuelled the disorder and 39 officers were injured. The political response by the Prime Minister, Sir Kier Starmer was to bring together the law enforcement agencies to work more collaboratively in a preventative approach to future incidents. He praised the police in his question-and-answer session (Sky News, 01/08/24, 16:14) acknowledging their resilience but also the difficulties they had faced in the traumatic scenes they had encountered. This is the nature of police work.

These incidents epitomise the working life of the police officer, moving from one traumatic incident to the next, exposed to scenes of death and mutilation and further in the future, reliving them in the recounting in statements, evidence gathering and evidence giving. This continues, case by case as the perpetrators enter the prison system and the risk assessments and supervisory work begins. The need for a better informed and trauma aware working environment for police, prison and probation officers is thus paramount; to their health, wellbeing and for some, their ability to do their role. These professionals are the key agencies that maintain the safety of our society, managing crime and criminals, and can be overlooked in terms of their own wellbeing and the issues caused by compassion fatigue. Moving from one traumatic incident to the next, one file to the next, revisiting imagery and supervising those who have experienced trauma, is part of their everyday working life yet, the mechanisms for support are limited and the effects largely ignored. Removal of informal debrief opportunities, high workloads that prevent the better allocation of traumatic cases, high sickness rates and austerity measures impacting on staff resources all play an integral factor to the day-to-day perpetuation of compassion fatigue.

Cultural issues are also problematic particularly within policing where the underlying masculinity of the organisation hinders the willingness of officers to admit to or seek help. But it also underpins those shared values to protect those in society who are perceived as 'weaker'. This is, in part, exacerbated by the raw media coverage that comes with bystander footage, often skewed and portraying the police in a negative light, criticising them for not responding in a way that the public feel that they should and portraying them in fictional dramas that supports this perception. The evident finger-pointing mentality that omits from the press both formal and informal can be damaging to all practitioners of these services; probation and prison officers are not exempt, and all are victims of the media blame culture so prevalent in British society.

The possibility of achieving a trauma-informed working environment within the criminal justice sector agencies is, therefore, fraught with obstacles, restrictions and cultural resistance. Nevertheless, the need is imperative.

References

Avon and Somerset Police Federation. (2021). Capture Data on Traumatic Incidents. Available from: https://www.polfed.org/avonsom/news/news-articles/capture-data-on-traumatic-incidents/. [Accessed 21 March 2024].

Beard, J. (2023). What is the Government doing to reduce pressure on prison capacity? *House of Commons Library* [online]. https://commonslibrary.parliament.uk/what-is-the-government-doing-to-reduce-pressure-on-prison-capacity/ [Accessed 13 June 2024].

Bristol North Somerset and South Gloucestershire. (2021). Principles for Trauma-informed Practice, Available from: https://bristolsafeguarding.org/media/rmlbpe2u/bnssg-principles-for-trauma-informed-practice-march-2021-web-version.pdf [Accessed 12 April 2024].

Burnett, M. E., Sheard, I., & St Clair-Thompson, H. (2020). The prevalence of compassion fatigue, compassion satisfaction and perceived stress, and their relationships with mental toughness, individual differences and number of self-care actions in a UK police force. *Police Practice and Research, 21*(4), 383–400.

Canton, R. (2011). *Probation: Working with offenders.* Routledge.

Clements, A. J., Sharples, A., & Kinman, G. (2021). Identifying well-being challenges and solutions in the police service: A World Café approach. *The Police Journal*, *94*(2), 81–101. [Accessed 21 March 2024].

Clements, A. J., & Kinman, G. (2023). Wellbeing in UK prison officers: Key factors. *Prison Service Journal*, *268*, 17–22. [Accessed 21 March 2024].

College of Policing. (2018). Responding to trauma in policing. A practical guide. Available from: https://assets.college.police.uk/s3fs-public/2021-02/responding-to-trauma-in-policing.pdf. [Accessed 12 April 2024].

Donovan, K. M., & Klahm, C. F. (2015) The role of entertainment media in perceptions of police use of force. *Criminal Justice and Behavior*, *42*(12), 1261–1281. [Accessed 1 June 2024].

Ellis, J. R. (2021). More than a trivial pursuit: Public order policing narratives and the 'social media test'. *Crime, Media, Culture*, *17*(2), 185–207. [Accessed 13 June 2024].

Foley, J., & Massey, K. L. D. (2021) The 'cost' of caring in policing: From burnout to PTSD in police officers in England and Wales. *The Police Journal, 94*(3), 298–315. [Accessed 1 November 2024].

Frost, L., & Scott, H. (2022). What is known about the secondary traumatization of staff working with offending populations? A review of the literature. *Traumatology*, *28*(1), 56–73. [Accessed 10 April 2024].

Graham-Kevan, N., Brooks, M., Willan, V. J., Lowe, M., Robinson, P., Khan, R., Irving, M., Karwacka, M., & Bruce, J. (2015). Repeat victimisation, retraumatisation and victim vulnerability. *The Open Criminology Journal*, *8*, 36–48. [Accessed 11 April 2024].

Grant, H. B., Lavery, C. F., & Decarlo, J. (2019). An exploratory study of police officers: Low compassion satisfaction and compassion fatigue. *Frontiers in Psychology, 9*, 1–5. https://doi.org/10.3389/fpsyg.2018.02793

Harper, C. A., Todd, E., Hogue, R., Bartels, M., Page, J., & Robertson, N. (2022). Extent and predictors of work-related distress in community correction officers: A systematic review. *Psychiatry, Psychology and Law, 29*(2), 155–182.

Harrison, K., & Nichols, H. (2023). The health and wellbeing of prison governors in England, Wales and Scotland, *Prison Service Journal* (268), 4–10.

Hilinski-Rosick, C. M., Branch, K. A., & Walker, A. (2023). Compassion fatigue among Criminology and Criminal Justice Interns. *Journal of Criminal Justice Education, 34*, 639–652.

HMPPS. (2020). Risk of Serious Harm Guidance 2020, Public Protection Group, v.3 Available from: https://assets.publishing.service.gov.uk/media/652cf8c9697260000dccf834/Risk_of_Serious_Harm_Guidance_v3.pdf

Jewkes, Y. (2011). *Media and crime* (2nd ed.). Sage Publications Ltd.

Kohm, S. (2009). Naming, shaming, and criminal justice: Mass-mediated humiliation as entertainment and punishment. *Crime Media Culture, 5*(2), 188–205.

Lewis, K. R., Lewis, L. S., & Garby, T. M. (2013) Surviving the trenches: The personal impact of the job on probation officers. *American Journal of Criminal Justice, 38*(1), 67–84. [Accessed 13 August 2024].

Maguire, L., & Sondhi, A. (2024). Stress-related psychosocial risk factors among police officers working on Rape and Serious Sexual Offences. *The Police Journal, 97*(1), 56–72. https://doi.org/10.1177/0032258X221128398

Manning, P. K. (1997) *Police work*. Waveland.

McCartan, K. (2022). Refining processes in policy and practice in working with people accused or convicted of a sexual offence. *HM Inspectorate of Probation Academic Insights 2022/01*, https://www.justiceinspectorates.gov.uk/hmiprobation/wp-content/uploads/sites/5/2022/01/Academic-Insights-McCartan.pdf

Memon, A., Hunt, A., Thelwall, E., Hardwick, N., & Johnson, S. U. (2023). The mental health of staff working in UK prisons during the Covid-19 pandemic. *The Howard Journal of Crime and Justice, 62*, 357–373.

Miller, J., Brewin, C., Soffia, M., Elliott-Davies, M., Burchell, B., & Peart, A. (2021). The development of a UK police traumatic events checklist. *The Police Journal, 95*(1), 207–223. https://doi.org/10.1177/0032258X211002597

MIND. (2023). Trauma. Available from: https://www.mind.org.uk/information-support/types-of-mental-health-problems/trauma/effects-of-trauma/ [Accessed 11 April 2024].

Ministry of Justice, HMPPS and Lord Timpson. (2024). Process activated to manage prisoner movements. https://www.gov.uk/government/news/process-activated-to-manage-prisoner-movements. [Accessed 29 June 2024].

Ministry of Justice. (2019). Her Majesty's Prison and Probation Service (HMPPS) workforce statistics bulletin, as at 30 June 2019. Available from: https-workforce-statistics-september-2019.pdf(publishing.service.gov.uk). [Accessed 29 June 2024].

Ogińska-Bulik, N., & Juczyński, Z., Burnout and posttraumatic stress symptoms in police officers exposed to traumatic events: the mediating role of ruminations. *International Archives of Occupational and Environmental Health, 94*(6), 1201–1209. [Accessed 11 April 2024].

Page, J., & Robertson, N. (2022). Extent and predictors of work-related distress in community correction officers: a systematic review. *Psychiatry, Psychology, and Law, 29*(2), 155–182. [Accessed 12 April 2024].

Papazoglou, K., & Tuttle, B. M. (2018). Fighting police trauma: Practical approaches to addressing psychological needs of officers. *Sage Open, 8*(3). [Accessed 2 May 2024].

Phillps, J., Westaby, C., & Fowler, A. (2020). Emotional labour in probation. *HM Inspectorate of Probation Academic Insights [online].* 2020/3, https://www.justiceinspectorates.gov.uk/hmiprobation/wp-content [Accessed 11 April 2024].

Phythian, R., Birdsall, N., Kirby, S., Cooper, E., Posner, Z., & Boulton, L. (2022). Developments in UK police wellbeing: A review of blue light wellbeing frameworks. *The Police Journal, 95*(1), 24–49. https://doi.org/10.1177/0032258X211073003

Rhineberger-Dunn, G., Mack, K. Y., & Baker, K. M. (2016). Secondary trauma among community corrections staff: An exploratory study. *Journal of Offender Rehabilitation, 55*(5), 293–307. [Accessed 28 June 2024].

Ricciardelli, R., Taylor, M., Maier, K., & Spencer, C. D. (2023). Parole work in Canada: Tensions in supervising people convicted of sex crimes. *International Journal of Offender Therapy and Comparative Criminology, 67*(16), 1699–1721. [Accessed 23 May 2024].

SAMHSA. (2014). Trauma-informed care in behavioural health services. *US Substance Abuse Mental Health Services Administration.* SAMHSA's Concept of Trauma and Guidance for a Trauma-Informed Approach. https://ncsacw.acf.hhs.gov/userfiles/files/SAMHSA_Trauma.pdf [Accessed 21 February 2024].

Senker, S., Eason, A., & McCartan, K. (in press). The nature of Trauma-informed Care in the treatment of men convicted of a sexual offence and a history of trauma. *Sex Offending: Theory, Research and Prevention.*

Senker, S. Eason, A., Pawson, C., & McCartan, K. (2023). Issues, challenges and opportunities for trauma-informed practice, *HM Inspectorate of Probation Academic Insights* 2023/10. https://www.justiceinspectorates.gov.uk/hmiprobation/wp-content/uploads/sites/5/2023/11/Academic-Insights-Senker-et-al-FINAL.pdf. [Accessed 12 December 2023].

Smith, L. (2023). Promoting staff wellbeing within HMPPS, and interview with Chris Jennings, Executive Director Wales for HMP Prison and Probation Service. *Prison Service Journal*, September 2023, No. 268.

Symmonds, T. (2023). Most probation services are over capacity, leaked data reveals, BBC News. 8 February 2023 https://www.bbc.co.uk/news/uk-64344284. [Accessed 21 February 2024].

Turner, A. (2023). Exploring police culture and reform strategies post charing cross: Insights from the literature. *Police Journal (Chichester), 96*(4), 593–610. [Accessed 13 April 2024].

University of Cambridge. (2024). The New Police Traumatic Events Checklist (PTEC). Available from: https://www.policingtrauma.sociology.cam.ac.uk/checklist. [Accessed 22 February 2024].

Uzieblo, K. (2024). Sexual abuse: The well-being of professionals: A shared responsibility [*ATSA Blog*]. Available from: https://blog.atsa.com/2024/03/the-well-being-of-professionals-shared.html. [Accessed 30 May 2024].

Violanti, J. M., Charles, L. E., McCanlies, E., Hartley, T. A., Baughman, P., Andrew, M. E., Fekedulegn, D., Ma, C. C., Mnatsakanova, A., & Burchfield, C. M. (2017). Police stressors and health: A state-of-the-art review. *Policing*, *40*(4), 645–656. [Accessed 21 February 2024].

Part IV

Community Integration, Harm Reduction and Desistence

12

Restorative Justice as a Response to Sexual Violence in England and Wales

Paul Gavin, Phil Cawley, Stephanie Kewley, Lol Burke, Nadia Wager, and Cody Porter

Introduction

Sexual violence is a global issue. It does not discriminate by age, race, ethnicity, or nationality, and it is a crime often motivated by power dynamics related to gender (Burns & Sinko, 2023). The World Health Organisation 'WHO' (2021) estimated that one in three of all women, approximately 736 million, are subjected to physical or sexual violence by an intimate partner or sexual violence from a non-partner, and this number has remained largely unchanged over the past decade. Women living in low and lower-middle-income countries are disproportionately

P. Gavin (✉) · C. Porter
University of the West of England, Bristol, England
e-mail: paul.gavin@uwe.ac.uk

P. Cawley · S. Kewley · L. Burke
John Moores University, Liverpool, England

N. Wager
Teeside University, Middlesbrough, England

K. McCartan et al. (eds.), *Developing and Implementing a Public Health and Criminological Approach to Tackling Sexual Abuse*, Palgrave Studies in Risk, Crime and Society, https://doi.org/10.1007/978-3-031-93634-0_12

affected, and an estimated 37% of women living in the poorest countries have experienced physical and/or sexual intimate partner violence in their life, with some of these countries having a prevalence as high as 50% (WHO, 2021). Victims/survivors often experience negative mental and physical effects because of the crime. They are often disempowered by both the offence and their pursuit of justice.

For a ten-year period, between March 2014 and March 2024, data from the Crime Survey for England and Wales (hereon in referred to as CSEW) show that there was an increase of 1.1% in the number of people aged 16 to 59 who were victims of some form of sexual assault (including attempted assaults). For the year ending June 2024, sexual offences increased by 1% (194,434 offences) compared with the previous year (192,432 offences). Approximately 36% (69,184 offences) of all sexual offences recorded by the police for that period were rape offences. This represented a 2% increase on the previous year ending June 2023 (67,903 offences). This follows a pattern of general increases in sexual offences over the last ten years, largely due to improvements in the recording practices of the police (Office for National Statistics, 2024).

Rape Crisis in England and Wales reports that six in seven rapes against women are carried out by someone they know, and one in two is carried out by a partner or ex-partner (Rape Crisis, 2024). They also report that of the 69,184 rapes recorded by the police in year ending June 2024, charges were only brought in 2.7%, or less than 3 in every 100 cases. Five in six women who are raped do not report it to the police and it can often be a hidden crime (Office for National Statistics, 2021). For those few who do go through the criminal justice system, many victims/survivors find it an extremely painful process (Burns & Sinko, 2023; Wheatcroft et al., 2009) as victims/survivors are "at every step of criminal proceedings…powerfully reminded of their marginal and dishonoured status" (Herman, 2005, p. 574).

Restorative justice (hereon in referred to as RJ) is not a new concept and is used internationally within criminal justice systems. There is a wide range of literature that traces its genesis and evolution from a response to crime to its integration into wider society as a general practice (Gavin et al., 2024a). While RJ is recognised as a suitable response to criminal offending, it has often proved controversial in the field of sexual violence (Daly, 2006, 2012) as it can be perceived as revictimising and even retraumatizing the victim/survivor (Marsh & Wager, 2015; McGlynn et al., 2012). Consequently, there is limited literature on the use of RJ in cases of sexual violence, and the limited use of RJ in such cases has often been met with criticism. The potential for revictimisation and retraumatisation, as well as the impact of power imbalances between the parties, are just some of the concerns that have been echoed (Gavin et al., 2024a, 2024b; Gavrielides, 2015).

This chapter examines the global research on the application of RJ in cases of sexual violence and then discusses how RJ has been developed for similar cases in England and Wales. It provides a critical analysis of some of the barriers to implementing RJ for cases of sexual violence in England and Wales; in particular, it considers the impact of COVID-19 and the development of the Restorative Practice Hub (Re-hub) in His Majestys' Prison and Probation Service (hereon in referred to as HMPPS). This chapter begins, however, with a brief discussion on whether we should be considering RJ, restorative practice or restorative principles.

Restorative Justice, Practice or Principles?

Although RJ has been a part of the criminological debate for decades, providing a universally agreed-upon definition of RJ continues to be elusive (Gavin & MacVean, 2018; Gavin et al., 2024a; Gavrielides, 2015). Marshall (1999, p. 5) provided a widely accepted definition of RJ as "a problem-solving approach to crime which involves the parties themselves and the community generally, in an active relationship with statutory agencies." The Council of Europe (2018, p. 3) states that RJ refers to "any process which enables those harmed by crime, and those responsible for that harm, if they freely consent, to participate actively in the resolution of matters arising from the offence, through the help of a trained and impartial third party". The range of definitions demonstrates that RJ remains all things to all people and perhaps should best be viewed as a suite of techniques or practices rather than a single prescribed approach (Gavin et al., 2024a).

The Restorative Justice Council (2016) identifies six principles of restorative practice: restoration, voluntarism, neutrality, safety, accessibility, and respect. This is to ensure that the primary aims are to restore harm, participants are taking part of their own free will, and the process remains unbiased, safe for expression, accessible and respectful. Restorative practice can thus be considered as a term used to describe principles, behaviours, and approaches which build and maintain healthy relationships and a sense of community to resolve difficulties and repair harm if there has been a conflict. The term restorative practice reframes some of the principles of RJ to be used in a more versatile way in environments other than the criminal justice system, for example in education (Payne et al., 2022) and healthcare settings (Drennan, 2018), where justice may not be required.

In the following section, we will explore the international literature on RJ in cases of sexual violence. However, it is important to acknowledge that all contributing authors are based in England and Wales, and the primary focus of this chapter is the development of RJ as a response to sexual violence within these jurisdictions. Therefore, we have chosen to adopt the definition provided by the Ministry of Justice (hereon in referred to as MOJ) (2015) for the purposes of our discussion:

> Restorative justice is a process that brings together individuals harmed by crime or conflict with those responsible for the harm, with the goal of finding a constructive path forward.

Restorative Justice in Cases of Sexual Violence: Reviewing the International Literature

In Canada, the Community Justice Initiative has run the *Revive* programme, a community-based sexual trauma support group, since 1982 (Community Justice Initiative website, n.d.). Using restorative principles, Revive provides a safe and confidential space for people convicted of a sexual offence to discuss their behaviour. An assessment of the programme (Rye et al., 2018) found that it helped foster victim/survivor empathy amongst its users, with participants recognizing the emotions of the victims/survivors as well as viewing the offence from the victim's/survivor's perspective. This allowed them to share expressions of remorse, regret, or guilt when describing their feelings towards the victim/survivor. While research has claimed that people convicted of a sexual offence often show very little concern for the impact of their actions, (Seto, 2005) it has been noted that feelings of shame and guilt, both of which can play a central role in the restorative process, can also help boost their empathy development (Hanson, 2003; Howells & Day, 2003; Greenwald & Harder, 1998).

In the United States, RESTORE (Responsibility and Equity for Sexual Transgressions Offering a Restorative Experience) was a community-based restorative conferencing project in Arizona that specialised in cases of adult sexual violence. It ran between 2003 and 2007 and used restorative conferencing through referrals from prosecutors. This was the first project to utilise both feminist and restorative principles to address the needs of victims/survivors in cases of sexual violence (Kasparian, 2014; Koss et al., 2003). An evaluation (Koss, 2014) of the programme assessed reasons for choosing the RESTORE programme, preparation and conference experiences, overall programme and justice satisfaction, and completion rates. Most victims/survivors wanted to hold the person convicted of a sexual offence accountable, while a majority of those convicted of a sexual offence felt that offering an apology to the victim/survivor was a major reason they chose to participate. Conferences were found to be positive, and participants felt safe, listened to, supported, and respected. All victims/survivors and their supporters felt satisfied or very satisfied with their preparation, the conference, and the agreed plan for redress. Despite its closure in 2007, it had a strong influence on the implementation of other programmes, particularly Project Restore in New Zealand.

The New Zealand-based Project Restore is a victim/survivor-led organisation that offers RJ to victims/survivors of sexual violence through conferencing, and occasionally, victim-offender mediation. Reasons for participation include victims/survivors wanting to hold the convicted person accountable for their actions by hearing how the offence had impacted them, wanting to have their voice heard and their story told, wanting an apology, and wanting some form of reparation (Jülich & Landon, 2013). Participants generally have been found to have a high regard for the process and appear, at least in part, "to have achieved some kind of healing" (Jülich et al., 2010, p. 48).

Daly's (2006) analysis of cases of youth sexual assault in Australia found that from the perspective of the victim/survivor, restorative conferences were better than the traditional court experience. The RJ process allowed the victim/survivor to confront the convicted person and make them aware of the impact the offending had on them. It also allowed the victim/survivor to challenge any denials or excuses that may have been offered. This was even more relevant as nearly half of the cases that went to court resulted in charges being dismissed, therefore, denying the victims any chance they may have had at obtaining justice. It was also found that the drawn-out court process, with its delays and adjournments, could end up victimising the victims. Some court cases took up to twice as long to conclude as conference cases, they shifted jurisdiction more often, and victims would have had to attend court an average of six times to learn the outcome of their case. For those who did appear in court, nearly half would find that the case was dismissed or withdrawn, again denying the victim any sense of justice being done. Daly et al. (2013) also found that there was a lower re-offending rate for those who completed a RJ conference than for those who went through the traditional court process. Another Australian study (Bolitho & Freeman, 2016) found that participation in RJ was very beneficial for the people who had been harmed where programmes met certain conditions. These conditions included providing safety and being responsive to their needs. Loff et al. (2019) found that eight out of ten victims/survivors of sexual violence said RJ should be made available to other victims/survivors. The mother of one participant said the process had enabled her daughter to move on with her life, as taking part in the process helped stop her daughter from committing suicide.

Klar-Chalamish and Peleg-Koriat (2021) examined how RJ was used in following cases of intra-familial sexual abuse in Israel. Six themes were identified from the data. These were: Initiation of the RJ process was due to a significant family milestone—which became a motivation to mend family relations; the process met participants' needs to repair the familial relationships to enable healing within the family unit; the family system was moulded into a place for healing and growth; the process met the needs of the victim/survivor who yearned for a voice and validation; the process enabled agreements on how the family would conduct themselves in the future; and the process was a turning point in the victim's/survivor's recovery journey. Overall, the study found that RJ had a significant role in repairing familial relationships and that victims/survivors and their wider family circle experienced a form of recovery. Participants described their RJ experience as "a turning point in their recovery process and as a platform for agreements on the victims' future conduct in the family space and regarding family relationships, all in a positive, future-facing approach that seeks to preserve those relationships" (Klar-Chalamish & Peleg-Koriat, 2021, p. 1065).

A review of the evidence suggests that RJ and its principles, when applied to cases of sexual violence, have generally been positive for victims/survivors who engage with restorative processes. Daly and Curtis-Fawley (2004, pp. 20–21) have stated that:

> a victim's account of the offence and its impact can be brought forward in a conference in a way not currently possible in court…the key source of victim validation and vindication is an offender's admission of wrong-doing…A case can only go to conference if an offender has made an admission…While such admissions may later be contested by the offender, they are checked and challenged by conference participants…This is the power of the conference process in cases of sexual assault.

Despite this, concerns remain. The European Forum for Restorative Justice (n.d.) has highlighted concerns over perceived leniency, power dynamics, victim/survivor safety, the potential for manipulation of the process by certain participants, pressure on victims/survivors, and conflicting loyalties, especially in terms of intra-familial sexual abuse. These concerns have resulted in a lack of RJ options for cases of sexual violence, and searches for studies or evaluations of RJ programmes for cases of sexual violence produce limited findings (Koss, 2014). Daly

(2012) has noted that in some cases the outcomes of the restorative process may appear too lenient. This might send the wrong message to potential participants. Using restorative processes could serve "to diminish the seriousness of the crime by demonstrating what might be perceived as a lenient or 'soft option' to the punishment of offenders" (Marsh & Wager, 2015, p. 340), especially in cases of child sex abuse (McAlinden, 2017).

There are also concerns over gender-based power dynamics, function safety, and accountability for wrong-doing when using RJ in cases of sexual violence. This is often due to the prevalence of the power imbalance during the offence, and the potential for the continuation and reinforcement of that imbalance during the RJ proceedings (Gavrielides, 2015; Jülich & Thorburn, 2017; Mercer et al., 2015). Power imbalances that go unchecked may reinforce violent behaviour and may compromise the safety of the victim/survivor. If managed incorrectly, the restorative process may present the potential for the continuation and reinforcement of that imbalance (Gavrielides, 2015; Jülich & Thorburn, 2017). This may lead to concerns over the safety of the victim/survivor in the process (Marsh & Wager, 2015). This relates to a further concern which is the potential for victims/survivors to be pressured or coerced into participating in the restorative process (Campbell et al., 2006; Daly, 2012; McCold & Watchel, 1998) and to accept outcome agreements or apologies (Stubbs, 2007). Any attempt to bring victims/survivors and those convicted of a sexual offence together when the victim/survivor's emotions are dominated by fear or anger may simply exacerbate their suffering (Wemmers & Canuto, 2002).

Manipulation of both the process and of the victim/survivor by certain participants is also a concern. This may be a result of the power imbalance between the parties and may lead to the revictimisation of the victim/survivor (Marsh & Wager, 2015). In cases of intra-familial sexual abuse, there may be mixed loyalties of family members, who may partly support victims/survivors, but also support those committing the offence, and may even collude with the violence (Cossins, 2008; Daly, 2006, 2012). This can be very confusing for some victims/survivors. In some cases, family members may blame the victims/survivors and treat them as being weak and vulnerable—such reactions can be a source of great distress and can be retraumatizing for victims/survivors (Klar-Chalamish & Peleg-Koriats, 2021).

The Use of Restorative Justice for Sexual Offences in England and Wales

Thames Valley Police are credited with pioneering RJ in the criminal justice system in England and Wales in the late 1990s with the application of RJ to the cautioning of young offenders (Davey, 2005). Since its inception, there has now been variance across England and Wales over who delivers RJ services. Initially, police forces following the Thames Valley lead, embraced RJ, but from 2013, the number of specialist services grew as Police and Crime Commissioners became responsible for funding RJ as part of their remit to commission victim services. From 2013 to 2016, the government provided earmarked (but did not ringfence) funding for RJ, including this in the overall victim funding allocation thereafter. As a result, in some police areas, Police and Crime Commissioners now provide and manage the service themselves; in others, RJ is commissioned externally on a competitive basis, with Remedi, Restorative Solutions, and Calm Mediation being some of the larger providers (Marder et al., 2023).

The growth of RJ has seen the development of guidance documents from the Association of Chief Police Officers (2012) and Restorative Justice Council (2020), that have highlighted, amongst other things, the circumstances and the offences for which it should be used. The MOJ have also published a series of action plans, beginning in 2012, the most recent iteration covering the period from November 2016 to March 2018. These plans had clear and ambitious goals, around 'quality' and 'awareness' of RJ with all victims having equal access to RJ at all stages of the criminal justice system (MOJ, 2017). However, whilst the Association of Chief Police Officers and Restorative Justice Council guidance recognise the use of RJ for offences of sexual violence, neither of these, nor the MOJ documents, are supported in legislation.

Despite fears of revictimisation and retraumatisation of victims/survivors, providers have engaged RJ for these offences but (despite a literature search) it is difficult to determine when RJ began to be used for cases involving sexual violence in England and Wales. This is also hindered by the lack of a centralised, or at least coordinated, approach to data collection. Whilst a study (Marsh & Wager, 2015) only found less than a handful of cases in the UK where victims/survivors had sought out and met the person who sexually offended against them in an RJ meeting, this would appear to be a starting point for its use. This is supported by the accounts of two victims/survivors around the same time who shared their own positive experiences of an RJ intervention in or on public platforms (Emma's Story, 2016; BBC News, 2014). Since this time, there has been a growing range of RJ interventions by RJ practitioners for a wide range of sexual violence offences (Cawley et al., 2023).

Increase in Restorative Justice Referrals

As publicity around the use of RJ for sexual violence has grown, agencies including HMPPS and victim services have begun to refer victims/survivors to RJ providers. In addition, RJ providers have actively sought to broaden referral pathways, in which agencies have responded positively, resulting in a proactive promotion of RJ in contexts such as witness care units and sexual offence victim/survivor projects. As a result, RJ practitioners can work closely with these agencies to deliver RJ interventions.

The Role of Police and Crime Commissioners and Commissioned Services in the Delivery of Restorative Justice

Police and Crime Commissioners[1] and commissioned services have embraced the use of RJ for sexually violent crimes, despite the increased

[1] Police and Crime Commissioners are elected in areas of England and Wales to make sure that local police meet the needs of the community. They are responsible for how areas are policed, the police budget, the amount of Council Tax charged for the police, the information you get about what the local police are doing, and, appointing and dismissing the chief constable (the

resources required to deliver RJ in these cases. RJ practitioners consider referrals on a case-by-case basis, individually risk assessing all referrals for which sexual violence is present. Commissioners have made additional resources available to providers to deliver RJ in cases of sexual violence, particularly because of the extra travel and training required (Cawley et al., 2023). RJ interventions generally take place in the area where the offence was committed, although this is not always possible as the person with the conviction may be serving a sentence of imprisonment out of the area, or the victim/survivor may have moved locality. These resources support practitioners travelling across England and Wales to meet potential participants and on as many occasions as necessary.

Budgetary provision has also been made available for practitioners to receive the basic level of training (a standardised 3-day package) from RJ training providers such as Remedi or Restorative Solutions. RJ practitioners receive additional training to enable them to deliver RJ in more serious and complex cases, including those for sexual violence. Providers have also sourced other specialised training, examples include specialist input on 'trauma informed approaches', input from Rape Crisis centre staff and input from staff who deliver the sexual offending behaviour programmes and interventions in the prison system. Whilst this training has begun to help improve the confidence of RJ practitioners, there remain some concerns in practice. Practitioners remain unclear about engaging and motivating people with sexual convictions to participate (Cawley et al., 2023). They lack the confidence to appropriately interpret body language, acts of coercion and control, and thus, rely heavily on the support of staff from other agencies, including prison psychologists, offender managers and counsellors (Gavin et al., 2024a).

Challenging the Fundamental Principles of Restorative Justice

The development of RJ for sexual violence in England and Wales since 2015 has seen RJ practitioners being prepared to 'challenge' some of

---

most senior police officer for the area). See https://www.electoralcommission.org.uk/voting-and-elections/how-elections-work/types-elections/police-and-crime-commissioners.

the basic tenets that RJ is built upon, and they may have adapted working practices as a result. For example, a person with a criminal conviction is required to accept responsibility before any RJ meeting can take place (Joyce-Wojtas & Keenan, 2016; Restorative Justice Council, 2020). This requirement is based on a belief that victims/survivors want to hear the person with the conviction accept responsibility for their behaviour, and that they would not want to engage with RJ otherwise. Whilst experience shows people who deny responsibility will unlikely engage in RJ, practitioners will still initiate the RJ process for victims/survivors while managing their expectations regarding the person with the conviction's intention to participate or not (Gavin et al., 2024a). Regardless if the person with the sexual conviction chooses to engage in RJ or not, the victim/survivor has agency and power over the decision-making process, ensuring their voice is heard and that their decisions are respected (Curtis-Fawley & Daly, 2005).

Furthermore, RJ interventions have generally been initiated by the victims/survivors of offences. Indeed some providers do not accept referrals from people with convictions (Banwell-Moore, 2023) as they believe their motivations to be disingenuous and risk revictimisation (Gavin et al., 2024a). However, a growing number of referrals initiated by the person convicted of a sexual offence are being made to RJ providers from police Management of Violent or Sexual Offender units[2] or Offender Managers in the community or custody. It is of concern that for those providers choosing not to take on these cases they are, albeit unintentionally, taking the decision-making process out of the hands of victims/survivors. This runs counter to RJ principles and as such, RJ practitioners who work for these providers have developed a 'workaround'. Where the victim/survivor is being supported by a victim/survivor supporting agency, on the RJ practitioner's behalf, the agency will talk in general about RJ with the victim/survivor and if they show any interest, the victim/survivor support agency will provide information which may result in the victim/survivor requesting RJ. This 'workaround' effectively results in the RJ process being victim/survivor-led (Gavin et al., 2024a).

---

[2] See https://www.college.police.uk/app/major-investigation-and-public-protection/managing-sexual-offenders-and-violent-offenders/introduction-managing-sexual-offenders-and-violent-offenders.

The Impact of the Restorative Practice Hub (Re:hub) and COVID-19

While the use of RJ for sexual offences continues to grow; two developments have impacted the delivery and practice of RJ for these cases. Firstly, the introduction of the Restorative Practice Hub (known as Re:hub) which was established in 2019 by HMPPS; the second challenge was COVID-19.

Re:hub was established to assure the quality and safety of restorative practice across the prison estate. It was introduced with little publicity about its role or purpose; this was planned for early 2020 and its initial introduction had little impact on RJ practitioners who continued to liaise directly with various agencies and prisons to progress RJ meetings. However, the arrival of the COVID-19 pandemic, which caused inevitable disruption to the delivery of RJ, also resulted in the postponement of the Re:hub launch with all visits to prisons suspended. Understandably, RJ was not a priority for prison governors who were struggling to contain the spread of COVID-19 within their establishments. RJ effectively came to a halt until around the second quarter of 2021 when visits to prisons recommenced (in a 'business as usual' way without COVID-19 restrictions) and RJ delivery returned to a degree of 'normality'. As COVID-19 restrictions eased, Re:hub became more proactive in controlling the process of RJ justice interventions. All potential RJ cases in prisons were required to be referred to the Re:hub to determine if cases could progress. This involved the establishment of multi-agency meetings between Re:hub staff, prison and probation staff and practitioners for each case. The initial impact of this change generated a considerable amount of work for Re:hub staff in establishing meetings. This resulted in what practitioners perceived to be unacceptable delays in cases being progressed. To overcome this, practitioners, where they could, continued to link directly with prisons that were not engaging with Re:hub and who were unaware of its role.

Almost four years after its inception, Restorative Practice Policy Framework guidance was issued in April 2023 providing greater clarity to HMPPS staff (and RJ practitioners) over Re:hub's purpose and operation. It contains guidance on the types of cases to be referred to Re:hub and in particular those that meet the criteria they have set, of being 'serious and complex'. It does not, however, give timescales for Re:hub to work to. Where prisons are risk averse to the concept of RJ conferences, practitioners are blocked from progressing these (Kirby & Jacobsen, 2015). A similar blockage has been experienced by RJ practitioners in England and Wales with the introduction of Re:hub in prisons.

Examples of Re:hub and HMPPS staff reaching decisions without consulting those with sexual convictions is problematic for both the person in prison, in that they are not provided with a choice to engage, but of perhaps greater concern, decisions are made in the absence of victim/survivors' consent. For a person in prison to make an informed decision on whether to engage in RJ, they must be made aware, at the very least, of who the victim/survivor is and their motivation for taking part. That the offer for RJ was made by the Prison Offender Manager who may have little knowledge of RJ is also problematic, as research suggests that the best person to explain and offer RJ to prospective participants is the person who will facilitate if they agree (Laxminarayan, 2014).

Discussion

The introduction of Re:hub has impacted RJ practitioners' capacity to deliver RJ for 'serious and complex' cases, especially in terms of the prolonged timescales they experience. Multi-agency meetings can be difficult to arrange because of the conflicting calendar arrangements of all those involved. For practitioners, this is a source of frustration as prior to the inception of Re:hub, via telephone calls, they could gather and disseminate all the information required to inform decision-making as to whether RJ should progress. Re:hub is arguably another 'gatekeeper' and 'hoop' that victims/survivors must jump through. As the Restorative Practice Policy Framework details timescales for Offender Managers and Victim Liaison Officers to fulfil their RJ obligations, it is disappointing that none have been included for Re:hub. This absence of timescales for the central processor of RJ continues to significantly hinder practitioners in their ability to work with and support victims/survivors and manage their expectations.

There remains a lack of public awareness of the availability of RJ, including for sexual offences. This is despite the publication of the Code of Practice for Victims of Crime in 2021 (Ministry of Justice, 2021). This outlines, firstly, the victim's 'right' to receive information about RJ following the report of a crime and secondly, how to access RJ services in their local area. Yet, the CSEW, found that only 5.5% of victims were offered an opportunity to participate in RJ in 2019/2020 (the last year for which figures are available), down from 8.7% in 2012/2013 (Office for National Statistics, 2021). Some police forces argue they make victims/survivors aware by fulfilling their obligations under the Code of Practice for Victims of Crime in differing ways including sending a letter about RJ with the crime number or sending a text to victims with the crime number and a link to further information (including detail on the RJ process). Nevertheless, greater effort is required from all service providers who have responsibility for meeting the rights of victims under the code at any stage of the criminal justice process to promote and make people aware of RJ options (Gavin et al., 2024a).

Despite the promotion of restorative interventions being rolled out across health, education, and social work contexts, a lack of public awareness is perhaps the biggest challenge to developing the use of RJ in England and Wales (Gavrielides, 2015). Each year RJ is promoted during International Restorative Justice Week, but this tends to be localised and at the discretion of those with an interest in RJ. Similarly, RJ providers promote RJ at other times of the year but again this tends to be localised and targeted, to victim services groups, probation, and within police forces (Gavin et al., 2024a). We are encouraged to note the issue of public awareness being addressed by the work of the Restorative Justice All-Party Parliamentary Group Inquiry into RJ, established in September 2021 in England and Wales. One of the recommendations (R3) from the Inquiry is for a new national action plan for RJ to be published by the MOJ and Home Office, which should include a specific communications plan (R8) to help raise public awareness of RJ. These plans would be overseen by a dedicated government minister (R9) who could lead the task of raising public awareness of RJ (All-Party Parliamentary Group on Restorative Justice, 2022).

Conclusion

This chapter has outlined the development of RJ as a response to sexual offending in England and Wales. International research (Daly, 2014; Gavin et al., 2024b; Joyce-Wojtas & Keenan, 2016; Julich & Landon, 2013; Koss, 2014; Marsh & Wager, 2015) has shown that RJ has an important role to play in terms of representing the voice and the views of victims/survivors, which might otherwise be sidelined in the traditional criminal justice process. While some progress has been made throughout England and Wales in the advancement of RJ as a response to sexual violence, there are still barriers in place. These include a lack of national direction, a lack of coordination, and a lack of a centralised approach to data collection. The Code of Practice for Victims of Crime has been a step forward in the right direction as have the recommendations of the Restorative Justice All-Party Parliamentary Group Inquiry. Going forward, it will be interesting to see whether these recommendations are fully implemented and if so, the potential impact that this may have on the development of RJ in England and Wales will have to be closely monitored. It would also be useful for research to be undertaken which can properly assess the impact of Re:hub on the delivery of RJ throughout the prison estate in England and Wales.

References

Association of Chief Police Officers. (2012). *Restorative justice and minimum guidance*. https://docslib.org/doc/9724893/acpo-restorative-justice-guidance-and-minimum-standards#google_vignette

All-Party Parliamentary Group on Restorative Justice. (2022). *RJ APPG inquiry into restorative practices in 2021/2022*. https://eprints.glos.ac.uk/10197/7/10197-Hobson-%282021%29-Restorative-justice-APPG-inquiry-into-restorative-practices.pdf

Banwell-Moore, R. (2023). Just an 'optional extra' in the 'victim toolkit'?: The culture, mechanisms and approaches of criminal justice organisations delivering restorative justice in England and Wales. *International Review of Victimology, 29*(2), 217–235.

BBC News. (2014). Rape Victim Meets attacker to forgive him. Retrieved January 9, 2014, from https://www.bbc.co.uk/news/uk-25666416

Bolitho, J., & Freeman, K. (2016). *The use and effectiveness of restorative justice in criminal justice systems following child sexual abuse or comparable harms.* Royal Commission into Institutional Responses to Child Sexual Abuse.

Burns, C. J., & Sinko, L. (2023). Restorative justice for survivors of sexual violence experienced in adulthood: a scoping review. *Trauma, Violence and Abuse, 24*(2), 340–354. https://doi.org/10.1177/15248380211029408

Campbell, C., Devlin, R., O'Mahony, D., Doak, J., Jackson, J., Corrigan, T., & McEvoy, K. (2006). *Evaluation of the Northern Ireland youth conferencing service.* Northern Ireland Office.

Cawley, P. A., Kewley, S., Burke, L., & Wager, N. (2023). Restorative justice for sexual violence offences in England and Wales: The challenges ahead. *Journal of Victimology and Victim Justice, 6*(2), 208–216. https://doi.org/10.1177/25166069231178573

Community Justice Initiative Website. (no date). https://cjiwr.com/cji-history-2/

Cossins, A. (2008). Restorative justice and child sex offences: The theory and the practice. *British Journal of Criminology, 48*(3), 359–378.

Council of Europe. (2018). Recommendation CM/Rec(2018)8 of the Committee of Ministers to member States concerning restorative justice in criminal matters. https://rm.coe.int/CoERMPublicCommonSearchServices/DisplayDCTMContent?documentId=09000016808e35f3

Curtis-Fawley, S., & Daly, K. (2005). Gendered violence and Restorative justice: The views of victim advocates. *Violence against Women, 11*(5), 603–638.

Daly, K. (2006). Restorative justice and sexual assault: An archival study of court and conference cases. *British Journal of Criminology, 46*(2), 334–356.

Daly, K. (2012). Conferences and gendered violence: Practices, politics, and evidence. In E. Zinsstag & I. Vanfraechem (Eds.), *Conferencing and RJ: International practices and perspectives.* Oxford University Press.

Daly, K. (2014). Reconceptualizing sexual victimization and justice. In I. Vanfraechem, A. Pemberton, & F. Ndahinda (Eds.), *Justice for victims: Perspectives on rights, transition and reconciliation.* Routledge.

Daly, K., Bouhours, B., Broadhurst, R., & Loh, N. (2013). Youth sex offending, recidivism and restorative justice: Comparing court and conference cases. *Australian and New Zealand Journal of Criminology, 46*(2), 241–267.

Daly, K., & Curtis-Fawley, S. (2004). *Justice for victims of sexual assault: court or conference?* https://www.griffith.edu.au/__data/assets/pdf_file/0019/226711/2006-Daly-and-Curtis-Fawley-Justice-for-victims-of-sexual-assault-pre-print.pdf

Davey, L. (2005). The development of restorative justice in the United Kingdom: A personal perspective. https://www.iirp.edu/images/pdf/au05_davey.pdf

Drennan, G. (2018). Restorative justice applications in mental health settings – pathways to recovery and restitution. In J. Adlam, T. Kluttig, & B. X. Lee (Eds.), *Violent states and creative states: From the global to the individual. Book II: Human violence and creative humanity*. Jessica Kingsley.

Emma's Story. (2016). Restorative justice council publication spring edition.

Electoral Commissions Website. (no date). Police and Crime Commissioners. https://www.electoralcommission.org.uk/voting-and-elections/how-elections-work/types-elections/police-and-crime-commissioners

European Forum for Restorative Justice. (no date). Restorative justice and sexual violence. https://www.euforumrj.org/en/restorative-justice-and-sexual-violence

Gavin, P., Kite, C., Porter, C., McCartan, K., & Cawley, P. (2024a). Restorative justice in cases of sexual violence: Current and future directions in the UK. *Contemporary Justice Review, 26*(4), 393–410.

Gavin, P., & MacVean, A. (2018). Police perceptions of restorative justice: Findings from a small-scale study. *Conflict Resolution Quarterly, 36*(2), 115–130.

Gavin, P., Wager, N., Palmer, J., Cawley, P., Walker, T., & Bates, A. (2024b). Restorative justice and harmful sexual behaviour (RJHSB): A commentary. *NOTA News, 95*(24), 28–32.

Gavrielides, T. (2015). Is restorative justice appropriate for domestic violence cases? *Revista De Asistenta Sociala, 4*, 105–121.

Greenwald, D., & Harder, D. (1998). Domains of shame: Evolutionary, cultural, and psychotherapeutic aspects. In P. Gilbert & B. Andrews (Eds.), *Shame: Interpersonal behavior, psychopathology, and culture*. Oxford University Press.

Hanson, R. K. (2003). Empathy deficits of sexual offenders: A conceptual model. *Journal of Sexual Aggression, 9*(1), 13–23. https://doi.org/10.1080/1355260031000137931

Herman, J. (2005). Justice from the victim's perspective. *Violence against Women, 11*(5), 571–602.

Howells, K., & Day, A. (2003). Readiness for anger management: Clinical and theoretical issues. *Clinical Psychology Review, 23*(2), 319–337.

Joyce-Wojtas, N., & Keenan, M. (2016). Is restorative justice for sexual crime compatible with various criminal justice systems? *Contemporary Justice Review, 19*(1), 43–68.

Jülich, S., Buttle, J., Cummins, C., & Freeborn, E. (2010). *Project restore: An exploratory study of restorative justice and sexual violence.* AUT University.

Jülich, S., & Landon, F. (2013). *Achieving outcomes for participants of project restore's restorative processes: The perspectives of participants.* Project Restore.

Jülich, S., & Thorburn, N. (2017). Sexual violence and substantive equality: Can restorative justice deliver? *Journal of Human Rights and Social Work, 2*(1), 34–44.

Kasparian, A. (2014). Justice beyond bars: Exploring the restorative justice alternative for victims of rape and sexual assault. *Suffolk Transnational Law Review, 37*(2), 377–410.

Kirby, A., & Jacobsen, J. (2015). *Evaluation of the pre-sentence restorative justice pathfinder*. https://core.ac.uk/download/pdf/141223924.pdf

Klar-Chalamish, C., & Peleg-Koriat, I. (2021). From trauma to recovery: Restorative justice conferencing in cases of adult survivors of intrafamilial sexual abuse. *Journal of Family Violence, 36*, 1057–1068.

Koss, M. (2014). The restore program of restorative justice for sex crimes: Vision, process, and outcomes. *Journal of Interpersonal Violence, 29*(9), 1623–1660.

Koss, M., Bacher, K., & Hopkins, C. (2003). Restorative justice for sexual violence: Repairing victims, building community, and holding offenders accountable. *Annals of the New York Academy of Science, 989*, 384–396.

Laxminarayan, M. (2014). *Accessibility and initiation of restorative justice.* European Forum for Restorative Justice.

Loff, B., Naylor, B., & Bishop, L. (2019). *Community-based, victim-centred restorative justice for sexual violence - A pilot.* Australian Institute of Criminology. https://www.aic.gov.au/sites/default/files/2020-05/CRG-33-14-15-Final-Report.pdf

Marder, I., Banwell-Moore, R., Hobson, J., & Payne, B. (2023). New ideas, enduring cultural barriers? An analysis of recommendations from the all-party parliamentary group on restorative justice in England and Wales. *Criminology and Criminal Justice*. https://doi.org/10.1177/17488958231198787

Marsh, F., & Wager, N. (2015). Restorative Justice in cases of sexual violence: Exploring the views of the public and survivors. *Probation Journal, 62*(4), 336–356.

Marshall, T. (1999). *Restorative justice: An overview*. Home Office.

McAlinden, A. M. (2017). Restorative justice and sex offending. In T. Sanders (Ed.), *The Oxford handbook of sex offences and sex offenders*. Oxford University Press.

McCold, P., & Wachtel, B. (1998). *Restorative policing experiment: The Bethlehem Pennsylvania police family group conferencing project*. Community Service Foundation.

McGlynn, C., Westmarland, N., & Godden, N. (2012). 'I Just Wanted Him to Hear Me': Sexual violence and the possibilities of restorative justice. *Journal of Law and Society, 39*(2), 213–240.

Mercer, V., Sten Madesen, K., Keenan, M., & Zinsstag, E. (2015). *Doing restorative justice in cases of sexual violence: A practice guide*. Leuven Institute of Criminology. https://researchrepository.ucd.ie/bitstream/10197/7160/4/SVandRJ_practiceguide_withcover_Sept2015.pdf

Ministry of Justice. (2012). *Restorative justice action plan for the criminal justice system*. assets.publishing.service.gov.uk/government/uploads/system/uploads/attachment_data/file/217311/restorative-justice-action-plan.pdf

Ministry of Justice. (2015). *Restorative justice action plan*. Ministry of Justice.

Ministry of Justice. (2017). *Restorative justice action plan for the criminal justice system for the period to March 2018 covering the period November 2016 to March 2018*. www.gov.uk/government/uploads/system/uploads/attachment_data/file/596354/rj-action-plan-to-march-2018.pdf

Ministry of Justice. (2021). *Code of practice for victims of crime in England and Wales (Victims' Code)*. https://www.gov.uk/government/publications/the-code-of-practice-for-victims-of-crime/code-of-practice-for-victims-of-crime-in-england-and-wales-victims-code

Office for National Statistics. (2021). *Nature of sexual assault by rape or penetration, England and Wales: Year ending March 2020*. https://www.ons.gov.uk/peoplepopulationandcommunity/crimeandjustice/articles/natureofsexualassaultbyrapeorpenetrationenglandandwales/yearendingmarch2020

Office for National Statistics. (2024). *Crime in England and Wales: Year ending June 2024*. https://www.ons.gov.uk/peoplepopulationandcommunity/crimeandjustice/bulletins/crimeinenglandandwales/yearendingjune2024#sexual-offences

Payne, B., Young, G., & Hobson, J. (2022). Expanding the use of restorative practices in schools in Northern Ireland. Towards an 'All School' Model. *Irish Probation Journal, 19*, 74–96.

Rape Crisis. (2024). *Rape and sexual assault statistics*. https://rapecrisis.org.uk/get-informed/statistics-sexual-violence/

Restorative Justice Council. (2016). *Forgive and forget?* https://restorativejustice.org.uk/blog/forgive-and-forget

Restorative Justice Council. (2020). Restorative practice guidance. https://restorativejustice.org.uk/sites/default/files/resources/files/Restorative%20Practice%20Guidance%202020_April%2020_0.pdf

Rye, B. J., Hovey, A., & Waye, L. (2018). Evaluation of a restorative justice based, community program for people who have offended sexually: Participant impact. *Contemporary Justice Review, 21*(3), 276–298.

Seto, M. (2005). Is more better? Combining actuarial risk scales to predict recidivism among adult sex offenders. *Psychological Assessment, 17*(2), 156–167.

Stubbs, J. (2007). Beyond apology? Domestic violence and critical questions for restorative justice. *Criminology and Criminal Justice, 7*(2), 169–187.

Wemmers, J. A., & Canuto, M. (2002). *Victims experiences with expectations and perceptions of restorative justice: A critical review of the literature*. https://www.justice.gc.ca/eng/rp-pr/cj-jp/victim/rr01_9/index.html

Wheatcroft, J., Wagstaff, G., & Moran, A. (2009). Revictimizing the victim? How rape victims experience the UK legal system. *Victims and Offenders, 4*(3), 265–284.

World Health Organisation. (2021). *Devastatingly pervasive: 1 in 3 women globally experience violence: Younger women among those most at risk*. https://www.who.int/news/item/09-03-2021-devastatingly-pervasive-1-in-3-women-globally-experience-violence

13

Employability Barriers for Those with a Sexual Conviction

Cody Porter and Hannah Merdian

Introduction

The journey towards employability for individuals who have committed sexual offences is laden with barriers and challenges. These individuals often face societal stigma, legal restrictions, and a lack of supportive resources, which collectively hinder their reintegration into the workforce. The UK faces unique challenges in supporting those with a criminal record to find employment. Rising levels of imprisonment have drawn attention to the difficulties people with a criminal record may face (Porter & McCartan, 2024). We have reached a crisis point for prison capacity, with more people than ever being incarcerated. In 2024, over

C. Porter (✉)
University of the West of England, Bristol, England
e-mail: cody.porter@uwe.ac.uk

H. Merdian
University of Lincoln, Lincoln, UK
e-mail: HMerdian@lincoln.ac.uk

K. McCartan et al. (eds.), *Developing and Implementing a Public Health and Criminological Approach to Tackling Sexual Abuse*, Palgrave Studies in Risk, Crime and Society, https://doi.org/10.1007/978-3-031-93634-0_13

twelve and a half million people living in the UK had a criminal record (Unlock, 2024).

This chapter explores these multifaceted obstacles through an Epidemiological Criminology 'EpiCrim' lens, examining the systemic and individual factors that contribute to the employability issues faced by this population. By understanding these barriers, we can develop more effective strategies to support their rehabilitation, aimed at ultimately reducing recidivism by fostering a safer and more inclusive society. In this chapter, we explore the positive aspects of employment for those with a criminal record before examining barriers faced by those with a sexual offence.

Employment Improves Well-Being

Meaningful employment is important for contributing to a person's life satisfaction and has been found to have positive outcomes (Waddell & Burton, 2016). From an economic perspective, employment provides financial stability for the individual and contributes to a functional society. This is because high employment rates contribute to societal well-being by reducing poverty and inequality, which in turn can lead to better public health outcomes.

Meaningful employment can enable individuals to meet their basic needs and pursue long-term goals, which enhances life satisfaction (Helliwell et al., 2023). Having a job provides a sense of purpose and boosts self-worth, both of which are strongly linked to higher happiness levels (Waller, 2020). This works because employment fosters social connections and a sense of community, essential for mental health and overall happiness. For many people, employment provides a sense of belonging, offering both structure and purpose, which can enhance confidence and self-esteem (Graffam et al., 2008; Millard et al., 2020). Being part of a workplace community can offer emotional support and a sense of belonging. Indeed, those who have access to employment report feeling happier and more content with their lives (Waller, 2020).

Conversely, when people cannot access or maintain employment, their health outcomes have been found to be less favourable. This is because, for instance, unemployment can negatively impact well-being, as it often leads to financial stress and a loss of social connections, resulting in lower happiness and life satisfaction (Helliwell et al., 2023). In addition to enhancing life satisfaction, employability has been found to reduce a person's likelihood of reoffending following a prison sentence (Willis et al., 2020), therefore presenting a meaningful contributor to the desistence process (Maruna, 2017; Willis et al., 2010).

Desistance and Employment

According to the desistance literature, for those with a criminal history, employment should provide greater benefits than offending (Becker, 1968; Maruna, 2017; Merton, 1938). This may be linked to the experience of employment creating greater social ties with the community (Sutherland & Cressey, 1978). As people begin to feel part of the community that they reside in, they are less likely to want to bring harm to it. Employment provides that sense of community connection and can help to encourage behavioural change (Uggen & Staff, 2001).

Desistance is both a behavioural aspect, encompassing the actual behaviour of refraining from criminal activity, and an ongoing process of identity transformation (Maruna, 2001). This process involves stopping criminal behaviour and adopting a new, non-criminal identity. For those with a sexual offence conviction, desistance is particularly challenging. The 'sex offender' label carries a unique and severe stigma that differentiates these individuals from those with other criminal records (Harris & Socia, 2016).

The sex offender label is difficult to break away from (Ricciardelli & Moir, 2013; Tewksbury, 2012). Individuals with an offending history are frequently perceived as being risky or untrustworthy (Denver & DeWitt, 2023; Lageson et al., 2015; Porter et al., 2023), and those with a sexual offence conviction are often viewed even more negatively (Cochran et al., 2020). This refl ects a broader issue: The stigma associated with sexual offences can lead to social isolation, limited employment opportunities, and ongoing discrimination, all of which has been found to hinder the desistance process (de Vries Robbé et al., 2015). Individuals labelled as sex offenders often face substantial barriers to reintegration into society, making it difficult for them to establish a new, healthy sense of identity. This societal rejection can perpetuate feelings of shame and hopelessness, which are counterproductive to desistance (de Vries Robbé et al., 2015; Willis et al., 2010). The transformation of identity is a gradual process that involves internalising new values and beliefs, often facilitated by supportive networks and opportunities for personal growth (Maruna, 2017).

On an individual level, the negative stigma surrounding criminal behaviour can further disrupt one's sense of purpose and belonging, especially where friends, employers, and family members are unwilling to fully accept someone with a criminal record (Gålnander, 2020; McNeill, 2006). Therefore, for desistance to occur, not only must individuals rewrite their self-narratives, but society must also allow space for those narratives to take hold (Maruna, 2001). Subsequently, it is important to create societal conditions that promote trust and mutual respect between those with a criminal past and society (McNeill, 2006).

Based on what is known about employability and offending, it is not surprising that studies have found that access to employment, even with short-term contracts, decreases a person's likelihood of reoffending (Blomberg et al., 2011; Kazemian et al., 2009; Uggen & Staff, 2001). Employment provides individuals with a sense of purpose and structure, which are crucial for maintaining a law-abiding lifestyle. Having a job helps to fill time that might otherwise be spent engaging in criminal activities, and it offers a legitimate means of earning an income, reducing the financial pressures that can lead to reoffending. Yet only 27% of prisoners in England and Wales find employment after release (Unlock, 2023).

The Relationship Between Reoffending and Employment

The relationship between reoffending and unemployment is complex. Nally and colleagues (2014) analysed post-release data from 6,561 individuals with a range of either violent, non-violent, sexual or drug offences. The authors found that education and post-release employment were significantly and statistically correlated with decreased recidivism, regardless of the offence classification. They also found a comparably higher unemployment rate among those who reoffended within the first year of release from prison. Accordingly, almost half of the recidivist offenders were re-incarcerated within 12 months of the initial release. While understanding the relationship with employment and reducing reoffending is complex, the limited evidence base appears to suggest a positive impact (Blomberg et al., 2011; Kazemian et al., 2009; Uggen & Staff, 2001). In summary, employment addresses a key criminogenic need because having a stable job provides financial stability, structure, and a sense of purpose, all of which are crucial contributors to maintaining an offence-free lifestyle.

Attitudes Towards "Sex Offenders"

Employment encourages desistance and enhances public safety (Harris, 2017; Lageson & Uggen, 2013). Yet despite the outlined societal benefits, many individuals with a criminal record struggle to successfully secure a job (Graffam et al., 2008; Harris, 2017; Mikkelson & Schweitzer, 2019). This is particularly difficult for individuals who have been convicted of a sexual offence (Tovey et al., 2022). Part of this is the public's distain for those individuals, which is difficult to change (Harris & Socia, 2016).

Individuals who have been convicted of a sexual offence face considerably more challenges than those with other convictions (Rydberg, 2018). They are less likely to be called to interview and are more likely to lose their jobs upon arrest (Agan & Starr, 2018; Pager, 2003). Part of the reason for this is linked to punitive public attitudes and the stigma that surrounds sexual offences (King & Roberts, 2017; Rogers & Ferguson, 2011).

Employer Attitudes

Ensuring a safe environment for both employees and customers is a priority for most managers who are responsible for making hiring decisions (Giguere & Dundes, 2002; Pager & Quillian, 2005), which has been confirmed in the experimental research into employment perceptions and decision-making (Porter et al., 2023, 2025a). As a result of this pressure, employers are often hesitant to hire individuals with a criminal record, and this hesitancy becomes magnified when a prior offence is sexual in nature (Harris et al., 2020; Haslewood-Pócsik et al., 2008).

Haslewood-Pócsik and colleagues (2008) asked employers in England to complete a questionnaire regarding their perspectives on hiring people with a criminal record. Noteworthy, 43% of the sample of 2500 respondents had some experience employing people with a prior offence either at the time of the research or in the past. They found that employers who had this experience were working across a range of industries such as in the voluntary, manufacturing, or health and care sectors. Most employers felt that the type of offence mattered for employment, and 70% of respondents stated they would not be willing to hire someone with a former sexual offence. The risk to staff (95%) and risk to customers (89%) were listed as the most common factors that dissuade employers from hiring those with a criminal history.

More recent research confirms these findings. A report, published by the Prison Reform Trust, highlighted stigma and barriers these individuals face in the job market. Through interviews and surveys with employers, the authors reveal a general reluctance to hire individuals with such convictions, driven by concerns about reputation, safety, and potential backlash from customers and staff (Harris et al., 2020). The report also discusses the importance of support and education for employers to help them understand the benefits of giving these individuals a second chance, emphasising the role of employment in reducing reoffending and aiding rehabilitation. These concerns were also consistent with Porter and colleagues' (2023, 2025a) studies that examined perceptions of employability using candidates with a sexual offence history. They found that when asking people to make hiring decisions after the disclosure of a sexual offence conviction, participants were concerned about public and staff safety, as well as the reputational damage they could encounter.

Legislation

In the UK, those with prior sexual convictions, like all other individuals with convictions, will be subject to the Rehabilitation of Offenders Act 1974. Under the terms of the Act, if an employer requests information about an applicant's criminal record, the applicant must provide this information unless the conviction has become 'spent'. Spent convictions are for crimes removed from a person's basic record. These tend to be less serious crimes that have resulted in a prison sentence that was less than two and a half years. This means that spent convictions will not come back on basic criminal record checks, and employees or recruits will not need to disclose spent convictions under the Rehabilitation of Offenders Act 1974.

In addition to this, the Multi-Agency Public Protection Arrangements (MAPPA) operate under the remit of the Criminal Justice Act 2003, which mandates the collaboration of various agencies, including the police, probation services, and social services, to manage the risks posed by sexual and violent offenders (Bryan & Doyle, 2013; Ministry of Justice, 2024a, 2024b) (for more information on MAPPA and its role in risk management please see Chapter 2). MAPPA teams conduct comprehensive risk assessments to determine whether individuals with a history of sexual offending should disclose their criminal convictions to prospective employers, even if not legally required under the Rehabilitation of Offenders Act 1974 (Ministry of Justice, 2024a, 2024b).

These decisions balance the individual's rehabilitation with the need to protect the community and vulnerable individuals. For instance, if a person with a history of sexual offending against a child applies for a role within a school setting, involving unsupervised access to children, the MAPPA team may require disclosure to ensure safety. Similarly, even if the job does not involve direct interaction with vulnerable populations, disclosure might still be necessary due to the sensitive nature of the data the person would have access to and the potential risk of misuse.

Additionally, under the Sexual Offences Act 2003 a range of restrictions can be imposed by means of a sexual offences prevention order (SOPO) based on the risk profile of the individual. These restrictions include prohibitions on individuals owning a computer or having access to the Internet. A SOPO may also restrict *what locations* an individual may visit, or *when* an individual may be outside their home. These restrictions may further limit employment opportunities, and in some cases may require a disclosure to gain flexible working contracts. It should be noted that these restrictions are not universal and instead are dependent on the perceived risk the individual poses to society.

Current Government Initiatives to Support Employment

Getting individuals with a criminal record into work a priority for His Majesty's Probation and Prison Service' (Ministry of Justice, 2023) and a key goal for practitioners within the Criminal Justice System (McGuire, 1999, 2013), which initiated a series of key strategies and employment-focused programmes, mostly within the prison service. These measures aim to break the cycle of reoffending by ensuring that individuals living in prison have the skills, support, and opportunities needed to secure stable employment and lead offence-free lives when they leave prison. Here are some key strategies and programmes:

1. **Employment Advisory Boards (EABs)**: These boards have been established in 92 prisons across the UK. Business leaders on these boards work with prisons to enhance education and training programmes, align them with local workforce needs, and improve the employability of prisoners upon release.
2. **Collaboration with Businesses**: Major companies have partnered with the government to recruit former prisoners. For example, Timpson, a UK-based retail service provider, is well-known for its commitment to hiring people with criminal records, offering them

roles in their stores and workshops. Virgin Trains has also partnered with the government to provide job opportunities for former prisoners, focusing on roles in customer service and maintenance.

3. **One-Stop Employment Hubs**: One-Stop Employment Hubs within prisons are primarily offered by HMPPS. These hubs are part of the New Futures Network (2025) initiative, which collaborates with various partners, including the Department for Work and Pensions, probation services, and education providers. These hubs are similar to job centres. They provide career advice, CV writing assistance, and other employment support services. The goal is to prepare people leaving prison for the job market and help them secure employment soon after release.
4. **Reducing Disclosure Periods**: The UK government has reformed the rehabilitation period for criminal records under the Police, Crime, Sentencing and Courts Act 2022, reducing the time that individuals with a criminal record must legally disclose their past convictions to potential employers. This change aims to remove barriers to employment for many individuals with criminal records. However, for those who have committed a sexual offence, stricter measures are in place to ensure public safety (Ministry of Justice, 2025). These include enhanced notification requirements, such as regular updates to the police, advance notification of contact with children or absences from their main residence, and prohibitions on changing names on official documents. These measures ensure that those with a sexual offence conviction are closely monitored to mitigate potential risks to the public.
5. **Work coaches and job fairs**: The Department for Work and Pensions employs Work Coaches who help former prisoners get job-ready through mock interviews and training. Additionally, the Prison Service hosts job fairs, connecting prison leavers with potential employers in sectors like hospitality, construction, and manufacturing.
6. **Specialised Training Programmes**: Programmes like the one run by DHL at HMP High Down provide individuals who are able to work with computers with hands-on experience in logistics and warehouse management, preparing them for employment upon release. Other

initiatives include coding and digital skills training to bridge the digital divide and enhance employment prospects in the technology sector.

7. **Release on Temporary Licence (ROTL):** This allows prisoners nearing the end of their sentences to work in community settings, further easing their transition back into society and increasing their chances of securing stable employment; those who do secure ROTL work appear more likely to enter employment upon release. For example, Hillier and Mews (2018) examined the impact of increased ROTL on reoffending rates. They found that individuals living in prisons who participated in ROTL were less likely to reoffend compared to those who did not. The report further highlighted that ROTL provides the individuals with valuable work experience, helped them build connections with potential employers, and supported their reintegration into the community. The findings suggest that ROTL can be an effective tool in reducing reoffending and improving post-release employment outcomes.

These strategies and programmes are aimed at supporting employment for individuals being released from prison. These initiatives are new and have not yet been evaluated. It is, however, possible that those with a prior sexual offence conviction will not benefit in the same way as those with other offence convictions.

Based on our collaborations (CP) with local prisons and third-sector organisations, we have heard anecdotal reports that staff are still struggling to find work opportunities or training programmes for those with a prior sexual offence conviction. These same difficulties are not reported when finding employment for individuals with other offence convictions. For example, Timpson, has a documented history of hiring individuals with criminal records, though it does not typically endorse hiring people with a sexual offence conviction (Inside Time Reports, 2024).

In summary, there are companies involved in broader efforts to support the employment of those with a criminal record. Still, those with a sexual offence are likely to find it more challenging to secure employment due to the nature of these convictions and the specific responsibilities associated with the certain roles.

Increased Criminal Record Checking

Over a five-year period (2018–2023), the number of criminal records checks has increased from 4.14 million to 7.54 million (Unlock, 2024). Unsurprisingly, 70% of employers admit to requesting information about a prior conviction upon application (Unlock, 2018). These questions often put employers off a candidate—before they have even met them. In addition, Unlock (2018) have found that when employers ask questions on the application form about prior convictions, they are written in a confusing or misleading manner. Finally, many employers who use this type of system do not call the candidate to the interview stage (Rovira, 2024). We also know from previous research on employment decision-making, that people are less likely to want to hire a candidate after a DBS is provided (Porter et al., 2023, 2025a). This is problematic for those with a criminal past trying to navigate the employment process.

Practitioner Perspectives

For practitioners, supporting the reintegration of individuals with a prior sexual offence conviction can be challenging. It is important to be able to identify employability barriers and to share best practice recommendations.

Circles of Support and Accountability (CoSA) is a community based quaternary prevention approach to the integration of people convicted of a sexual offence whereby members of the community support the core member (i.e., person convicted of a sexual offence) with harm reduction through poor social modelling and supportive practices (McCartan & Kemshall, 2023). In 2024, we asked Circles volunteers how important employment was for them when working with a core member. Most volunteers felt they needed more training on advising their core members, particularly when to disclose their offences to employers. Interestingly, these findings were also reflected in a NOTA[1] 2024 conference workshop that we conducted with practitioners (CP & KMcC). The workshop highlighted that practitioners were struggling with the psychological impacts of working with this group. These frustrations were largely due to the stigma associated with the 'sex offender' label which made finding employment opportunities challenging. Many practitioners talked about how they used their own personal connections to support people with a prior sexual offence conviction to find employment. Practitioners reported challenges in supporting these individuals, noting the ineffectiveness of generic initiatives like "Ban the Box" and the difficulties in finding meaningful employment. The workshop recommendations were based on practitioners' frustrations with punitive risk management systems and the lack of standardised guidance. The findings highlight the importance of tailored approaches to improve employability and reintegration, advocating for more research and policy development. Finally, the evaluation of Circles ReBoot, a Circles progamme targeted at individuals convicted on online child sexual offending against children, highlighted education and employment as core needs of the attendees even after completion of the programme (Bradshaw et al., 2023).

Some agencies and legal advisors have guidelines on whether employers must work with those convicted of a sexual offence. *Employers Direct* argues that you may be able to dismiss an employee under reputation damage. They explain that employers cannot make unproven claims simply because an employee has been charged or convicted, but they could dismiss for reputational damage. On their webpage, they even provide an example stating, "*…you would need to prove that customers are withdrawing contracts or refusing to work with them because of the offence*". Knowing when to disclose a prior offence can be difficult, and people with criminal records vary in their approaches, with some individuals wanting to be open and honest, while others try to avoid the topic (Lindsay, 2022).

[1] NOTA is the National Organisation for the Treatment of Abuse, which includes multidisciplinary membership comprised of practitioners, managers and policy makers from the public, private and voluntary sectors.

Disclosure and Barring Services (DBS)

There are many barriers for those obtaining employment with a previous conviction. Disclosure and barring services (DBS) checks, as well as negative public opinion, contribute to this difficulty (Denver et al., 2017; Fletcher, 2004; Lukies et al., 2011; Porter et al., 2023). Legally there will be instances when a person must disclose their prior offence. However, even when an individual is better suited and more skilled than other candidates, employers are often less willing to hire the candidate when their criminal conviction is revealed (Lukies et al., 2011; Porter et al., 2023). One attempt to address this is through the ban the box initiative.

Ban the Box

The 'Ban the Box' law has been introduced in 35 states in the United States (Avery & Hernandez, 2019) and is becoming more popular in the UK. 'Ban the Box' removes the requirement to declare a prior conviction at the application stage and to allow the candidate to demonstrate that they meet the job requirements. As part of the 'Ban the Box' campaign employers will not ask applicants to tick a box about their criminal history in the initial stages of recruitment. This information is instead requested later in the hiring process. The idea is that applicants will be assessed on their qualifications and experience (without employers' pre-judgement regarding their criminal record). The objective is to ensure that employers have access to all relevant information to make their assessments. Porter et al. (2023, 2025a) investigated whether participants will change their initial hiring decision after a DBS check. This allows us to gain an understanding of how often people may reject a candidate on the sole grounds of their prior conviction.

In theory, this should mean that when a candidate is selected, the employer is more invested in hiring them, despite their prior offence. However, there is limited research on this. Additionally, we know that those with a sex-based criminal offence are perceived more negatively than other types of offenders. In this case, it may actually be harmful to not disclose a prior sexual offence. In Porter et al.'s (2023, 2025a) study, they found that participants no longer wished to hire the candidate they selected after the DBS revealed a prior sexual offence. Most participants felt that not disclosing this offence at the CV or interview stage was problematic, and made the candidate seem untrustworthy.

Mitigating Risk

Individuals making hiring decisions frequently report feeling that their business or company is at risk when a candidate has a prior sexual offence. This risk includes the physical risk that a person with a prior sexual offence history might pose to their staff (Porter et al., 2023) or the reputation risk that might occur if members of the public find out that a former offender has been hired (Porter et al., 2023, 2025a). Practitioners often disclose that when they work with employers a key concern is the reputational risk.

Mitigating risk is challenging. Some practitioners have found that when they highlight the fact that the authorises are aware of this person because of their prior offences, it helps. Although these practitioner reflections are useful for helping us to learn more about what works, there has been little empirical evidence to support this. Another potential way to mitigate this risk is by providing a support letter highlighting the positive characteristics or by verbally endorsing the individual. Some practitioners have reflected this recommendation through insights we collected at the NOTA conference. Interestingly, this appears effective when practitioners use their own personal connections. Of course, not all practitioners will have personal connections they can use to support their clients.

In terms of academic literature, there is a lack of this, especially in the UK. However, there is some evidence to suggest that reference letters can improve general employability within the labour market (Abel et al., 2020). In relation to employability and criminal records, Denver and DeWitt (2023) found increased employer trust when the candidate with a previous conviction provided a reference letter that highlighted desirable skills such as productivity, motivation, and trustworthiness. Giguere and Dundes (2002) also found individuals were more likely to hire a former offender if they were described as having a good work ethic and personal qualities. This suggests that the endorsement of another individual can increase the likelihood of being hired (DeWitt & Denver, 2020; Hunt et al., 2018). While these findings were from samples based in the USA, Porter and colleagues are examining the use of a support letter from probation and Circles UK in two different empirical studies, which appear to increase employment. This is particularly effective for those with child-based sexual offences or internet-based sexual offence histories.

More research is needed to help us understand why employers make decisions to hire or reject a candidate with a prior sexual offence history. While we have definitive support for employment as a protective factor for reducing reoffending, we cannot have the same level of confidence in our understanding of employer decision-making. Most of the work on sexual offending and employability has been conducted within the specific context of the US and with less scientifically robust research (Porter et al., 2025b).

Conclusion

This chapter has explored employability barriers and challenges for those who sexually offend, has highlighted some of the employment programmes and other support offer available, and has reviewed the empirical literature on this topic. This appears to be an area where more development is needed, and we call on practitioners working in the reintegration field to consider employment, work-related aspirations, and education as part of the reintegration plan. Prolonged periods of unemployment can lead to depression, anxiety, and a low sense of self-worth (Helliwell et al., 2023) and increasing access to education enhances employability and may support people to improve their well-being.

References

Abel, M., Burger, R., & Piraino, P. (2020). The value of reference letters: Experimental evidence from south Africa. *American Economic Journal: Applied Economics, 12*(3), 40–71. https://doi.org/10.1257/app.20180666

Agan, A., & Starr, S. (2018). Ban the box, criminal records, and racial discrimination: A field experiment. *The Quarterly Journal of Economics, 133*(1), 191–235. https://doi.org/10.1093/qje/qjx028

Avery, B., & Hernandez, P. (2019). Ban the box: US cities, counties, and states adopt fair-chance policies to advance employment opportunities for people with past convictions. National employment law project.

Becker, G. S. (1968). Crime and punishment: An economic approach. In *The economic dimensions of crime* (pp. 13–68). Palgrave Macmillan.

Blomberg, T., Bales, W., Mann, K., Piquero, A., & Berk, R. (2011). Incarceration, education and transition from delinquency. *Journal of Criminal Justice, 39*(4), Article 355365. https://doi.org/10.1016/j.jcrimjus.2011.04.003

Bradshaw, H. K., Perkins, D., & Merdian, H. L. (2023). *Findings from a feasibility study on circles ReBoot*. Circles UK.

Bryan, T., & Doyle, P. (2013). Developing multi-agency public protection arrangements. In *Sex offenders in the community* (pp. 189–206). Willan.

Cochran, J., Toman, E., Shields, R., & Mears, D. (2020). A uniquely punitive turn? Sex offenders and the persistence of punitive sanctioning. *Journal of Research in Crime and Delinquency, 58*(1), 74–118. https://doi.org/10.1177/0022427820941172

Course. In C. Gibson & M. Krohn (Eds.), *Handbook of life-course criminology* (pp. 201–212). Springer. https://doi.org/10.1007/978-1-4614-5113-6_12

de Vries Robbé, M., Mann, R. E., Maruna, S., & Thornton, D. (2015). An exploration of protective factors supporting desistance from sexual offending. *Sexual Abuse, 27*(1), 16–33. https://doi.org/10.1177/1079063214547582

Denver, M., & DeWitt, S. E. (2023). "[It's] what you do after the mistake that counts": Positive employment credentials, criminal record stigma, and potential pathways of mediation. *Criminology, 61*(1), 5–39. https://doi.org/10.1111/1745-9125.12319

Denver, M., Siwach, G., & Bushway, S. (2017). A new look at the employment and recidivism relationship through the lens of a criminal background check. *Criminology, 55*(1), 174–204. https://doi.org/10.1111/1745-9125.12130

DeWitt, S. E., & Denver, M. (2020). Criminal records, positive employment credentials, and race. *Journal of Research in Crime and Delinquency, 57*(3), 333–368. https://doi.org/10.1177/0022427819886111

Fletcher, D. (2004). *Reducing re-offending: The enterprise option.* Centre for Regional Economic and Social Research. https://shura.shu.ac.uk/27105/1/reducing-reoffending-enterprise-option.pdf

Gålnander, R. (2020). 'Shark in the Fish Tank': Secrets and stigma in relational desistance from crime. *The British Journal of Criminology, 60*(5), 1302–1319. https://doi.org/10.1093/bjc/azaa015

Giguere, R., & Dundes, L. (2002). Help wanted: A survey of employer concerns about hiring exconvicts. *Criminal Justice Policy Review, 13*(4), 396–408. https://doi.org/10.1177/088740302237806

Graffam, J., Shinkfield, A. J., & Hardcastle, L. (2008). The perceived employability of ex-prisoners and offenders. *International Journal of Offender Therapy and Comparative Criminology, 52*(6), 673–685. https://doi.org/10.1177/0306624X07307783

Harris, A. J., & Socia, K. M. (2016). What's in a name? Evaluating the effects of the "sex offender" label on public opinions and beliefs. *Sexual Abuse, 28*(7), 660–678. https://doi.org/10.1177/1079063214564391

Harris, D. (2017). *Desistance from sexual offending: Narratives of retirement.* Palgrave MacMillan. https://doi.org/10.1007/978-3-319-63200-1

Harris, M., Tynan, R., & Edgar, K. (2020). Thinking differently: Employers views on hiring people convicted of sexual offences. *Prison Reform Trust.* Retrieved from https://prisonreformtrust.org.uk/wpcontent/uploads/old_files/Documents/Thinking%20differently_web.pdf

Haslewood-Pócsik, I., Brown, S., & Spencer, J. (2008). A not so well-lit path: Employers' perspectives on employing ex-offenders. *The Howard Journal of Criminal Justice, 47*(1), 18–30. https://doi.org/10.1111/j.1468-2311.2008.00501.x

Helliwell, J. F., Layard, R., & Sachs, J. (2023). *World happiness report 2023.* Sustainable Development Solutions Network. https://worldhappiness.report/

Hillier, J., & Mews, A. (2018). *The reoffending impact of increased release of prisoners on Temporary Licence.* Ministry of Justice. Retrieved from https://assets.publishing.service.gov.uk/government/uploads/system/uploads/attachment_data/file/709123/rotl-report.pdf

Hunt, P., Smart, R., Jonsson, L., & Tsang, F. (2018). Breaking down barriers: Experiments into policies that might incentivize employers to hire ex-offenders. *RAND Corporation.* https://doi.org/10.7249/RR2142

Inside Time Reports. (2024, December 4). Timpson: I don't know how to rehabilitate sex offenders. Inside Time. Retrieved from https://insidetime.org/newsround/timpson-i-dont-know-how-to-rehabilitate-sex-offenders/

Kazemian, L., Farrington, D. P., & Le Blanc, M. (2009). Can we make accurate long-term predictions about patterns of de-escalation in offending behavior? *Journal of Youth and Adolescence, 38*, 384–400.

King, L. L., & Roberts, J. J. (2017). The complexity of public attitudes toward sex crimes. *Victims & Offenders, 12*(1), 71–89. https://doi-org.ezproxy.uwe.ac.uk/https://doi.org/10.1080/15564886.2015.1005266

Lageson, S., & Uggen, C. (2013). How work affects crime—And crime affects work—Over the life

Lindsay, S. L. (2022). Damned if you do, damned if you don't: How formerly incarcerated men navigate the labor market with prison credentials. *Criminology, 60*(3), 455–479. https://org.ezproxy.uwe.ac.uk/https://doi.org/10.1111/1745-9125.12307

Lukies, J., Graffam, J., & Shinkfield, A. J. (2011). The effect of organisational context variables on employer attitudes toward employability of ex-offenders. *International Journal of Offender Therapy and Comparative Criminology, 55*(3), 460–475.

Maruna, S. (2001). Making good: How ex-convicts reform and rebuild their lives. *American Psychological Association.* https://doi.org/10.1037/10430-000

Maruna, S. (2017). Going straight: Desistance from crime and life narratives of reform. In *The termination of criminal careers* (pp. 175–210). Routledge.

McCartan, K., & Kemshall, H. (2023). Incorporating quaternary prevention: Understanding the full scope of public health practices in sexual abuse prevention. *International Journal of Offender Therapy and Comparative Criminology, 67*(2–3), 224–246. https://doi.org/10.1177/0306624X211049204.

McGuire, J. (2013). "What works" to reduce re-offending: 18 years on. In L. A. Craig, L. Dixon & T. A. Gannon (Eds.), *What works in offender rehabilitation: An evidence-based approach to assessment and treatment* (pp. 20–49). Wiley Blackwell. https://doi.org/10.1002/9781118320655.ch2

McGuire, J. (Ed.). (1999). *What works: Reducing reoffending guidelines from research and practice* (Vol. 7). Wiley.

McNeill, F. (2006). A desistance paradigm for offender management. *Criminology and Criminal Justice, 6*(1), 39–62. https://doi.org/10.1177/1748895806060666

Merton, R. K. (1938). Social structure and anomie. *American Sociological Review, 3*(5), 672–682. https://doi.org/10.2307/2084686

Mikkelson, S., & Schweitzer, K. (2019). Hiring the formerly incarcerated: The mediating role of morality. *Criminal Justice and Behaviour, 46*(12), 1757–1774.

Millard, L., Hollins, N., & Sharman, R. (2020). Students as colleagues: Creating belonging and confidence through employment on campus. In W. Ashall & W. Garnham (Eds.), *Transitions into, through and out of higher education: Supporting students* (pp. 17–19). Staff and Educational Development Association. https://rke.abertay.ac.uk/ws/portalfiles/portal/31742596/Millard_StudentsAsColleagues_Accept ed_2020.pdf

Ministry of Justice. (2023). *Regional reducing reoffending plans: Annual update 2023*. https://www.gov.uk/government/publications/regional-reducing-reoffending-plans

Ministry of Justice (2024a). Prison population figures. Gov.UK. Retrieved from https://www.gov.uk/government/publications/prison-population-figures-2024

Ministry of Justice. (2024b). *Multi-agency public protection arrangements (MAPPA): Guidance*. Retrieved from https://www.gov.uk/government/publications/multi-agency-public-protection-arrangements-mappa-guidance

Ministry of Justice. (2025). *Crime and policing bill 2025: Management of offenders factsheet*. Retrieved from https://www.gov.uk/government/publications/crime-and-policing-bill-2025-factsheets/crime-and-policing-bill-management-of-offenders-factsheet

Nally, J., Lockwood, S., Ho, T., & Knutson, K. (2014). Post-release recidivism and employment among different types of released offenders: A 5-year follow-up study in the United States. *International Journal of Criminal Justice Sciences, 9*(1), 16.

New Futures Network. (n.d.). *Employment hubs*. Retrieved March 6, 2025, from https://newfuturesnetwork.gov.uk/employment-hubs/

Pager, D. (2003). The mark of a criminal record. *American Journal of Sociology, 108*(5), 937–975. https://doi.org/10.1086/374403

Pager, D., & Quillian, L. (2005). Walking the talk? What employers say versus what they do. *American Sociological Review, 70*(3), 355–380. https://doi.org/10.1177/000312240507000

Porter, C. N, Haggar, L., & Harvey, A. (2023). Sexual offending and barriers to employability: Public perceptions of who to hire. *Current Psychology, 42*, 28799–28811.

Porter, C. N., Haggar, L., Harvey, A. C., & Gavin, P. (2025a). Sexual misconduct and evaluation of candidate appropriateness for employment within a nonpublic-facing role. *International Journal of Law, Crime and Justice, 80*, 100721.

Porter, C. N., Gavin, P., Merdian, H., & Zloteanu, M. (2025b). Exploring social perceptions of hiring individuals convicted of sexual offences in the United Kingdom: A methodological review. *Journal of Criminal Psychology*. https://doi.org/10.1108/JCP-10-2024-0101

Ricciardelli, R., & Moir, M. (2013). Stigmatized among the stigmatized: Sex offenders in Canadian penitentiaries. *Canadian Journal of Criminology and Criminal Justice, 55*(3), 353–385. https://doi.org/10.3138/cjccj.2012.E22

Rogers, D. L., & Ferguson, C. J. (2011). Punishment and rehabilitation attitudes toward sex offenders versus nonsexual offenders. *Journal of Aggression, Maltreatment & Trauma, 20*(4), 395–414. https://doi-org.ezproxy.uwe.ac.uk/https://doi.org/10.1080/10926771.2011.570287

Rovira, M. (2024). Invisible stripes? A field experiment on the disclosure of a criminal record in the British labour market and the potential effects of introducing ban-the-box policies. *The British Journal of Criminology, 64*(4), 827–845. https://doi.org/10.1093/bjc/azad063

Rydberg, J. (2018). Employment and housing challenges experienced by sex offenders during re-entry on parole. *Corrections, 3*(1), 15–37. https://org.ezproxy.uwe.ac.uk/https://doi.org/10.1080/23774657.2017.1369373

Tewksbury, R. (2012). Stigmatization of sex offenders. *Deviant Behavior, 33*(8), 606–623. https://doi.org/10.1080/01639625.2011.636690

Tovey, L., Winder, B., & Blagden, N. (2022). 'It's ok if you were in for robbery or murder, but sex offending, that's a no no': A qualitative analysis of the experiences of 12 men with sexual convictions seeking employment. *Psychology, Crime & Law, 29*(6), 653–676. https://doi.org/10.1080/1068316X.2022.2030736

Uggen, C., & Staff, J. (2001). Work as a turning point for criminal offenders. *Corrections Management Quarterly, 5*(4), 1–16.

Unlock. (2018). A question of fairness: Research into employers asking about criminal records at application stage. Retrieved form https://unlock.org.uk//wp-content/uploads/misc/A-question-of-fairness.pdf

Unlock. (2024). New figures confirm more than 12.5 million people in the UK have a criminal record. Retrieved from https://unlock.org.uk/new-figures-confirm-more-than-12-5-million-people-in-the-uk-have-a-criminal-record/#:~:text=The%20Home%20Office%20have%20confirmed,(PNC)%20in%20April%202024.

Waddell, G., & Burton, A. (2016). *Is work good for your health and well-being? An independent review*. Department for Work and Pensions. https://assets.publishing.service.gov.uk/media/5a7cd68640f0b6629523c1de/hwwb-is-workgood-for-you-exec-summ.pdf

Waller, L. (2020). Fostering a sense of belonging in the workplace: Enhancing well-being and a positive and coherent sense of self. In *The Palgrave handbook of workplace well-being* (pp. 1–27).

Willis, G. M., Kelley, S. M., & Thornton, D. (2020). Are protective factors valid constructs? Interrater reliability and construct validity of proposed protective factors against sexual reoffending. *Criminal Justice and Behavior, 47*(11), 1448–1467. https://doi.org/10.1177/0093854820941039

Willis, G. M., Levenson, J. S., & Ward, T. (2010). Desistance and attitudes towards sex offenders: Facilitation or hindrance? *Journal of Family Violence, 25*(6), 545–556. https://doi.org/10.1007/s10896-010-9314-8

Part V

Conclusion and Future Directions

14

Where Next for EpiCrim Approaches to Understanding, Responding to and Preventing Sexual Abuse

Kieran McCartan

Introduction

The aim of this book was to better understand the challenges and opportunities of an Epidemiological Criminology (EpiCrim) approach to the prevention of sexual abuse. The book has reinforced that although there is political and academic agreement that sexual abuse is preventable, this has not historically translated into policy transformation, practice development or research investment (Brown, 2017; ECPAT international, 2024; King-Hill, 2022). In understanding the historical and current state of EpiCrim approach to sexual abuse, the book will end with a discussion of what happens next in the area and how the field could progress and develop in the next 10–20 years. The book concludes presenting the main outcomes/issues discussed with opportunities for future developments and recommendations highlighted.

K. McCartan (✉)
University of the West of England, Bristol, England
e-mail: kieran.mccartan@uwe.ac.uk

K. McCartan et al. (eds.), *Developing and Implementing a Public Health and Criminological Approach to Tackling Sexual Abuse*, Palgrave Studies in Risk, Crime and Society, https://doi.org/10.1007/978-3-031-93634-0_14

Overarching Findings from the Book

Section One: Concept, Context, and Evaluation Frames

Section one is a discussion of the theory, practice and evidence base of the EpiCrim approach. The section starts with a discussion of what EpiCrim is and how it relates to research, policy and practice in the field of sexual abuse. **McCartan and King-Hill** (Chapter 2) emphases that there is a political, policy, and practice willingness to engage in public health-based approaches to the prevention and response to all forms of sexual abuse, but that the evidence base is not as robust, and therefore it did not often provide academic cover to professionals in implementing these policies. Which is evident in the following chapter by **Kemshall** (Chapter 3) which highlights the opportunities and challenges of implementing a public health approach into an already established and developed criminal justice system. Kemshall argues that for multi-agency and multi-disciplinary working to flourish there needs to be shared values, shared language, shared platforms, and co-ordinated working in frontline professional services, which exists (i.e. MAPPA) but needs to be built on and effectively measured. This dovetails neatly with Green and **Richie** (Chapter 4) who argue that the research and evidence base around EpiCrim approaches needs to develop more to enable socio-political change and mainstream sexual abuse prevention. Richie and Green argue that there needs to be clear, streamlined and fit for purpose Key Performance Indictors for EpiCrim approaches. These do not currently exist, as the current datasets unsuccessfully try to bridge psychology, criminology, policy, and health databases. This means that the data is incomplete, poorly constructed and not able to talk to the theoretical, policy and practice outcomes needed to evidence EpiCrim, all of which often account for and measure different outcomes. The chapter offers insights into the challenges of doing socially sensitive research before offering solutions based on the five safes model of data collection and integrity.

The main finding from section one is that ***there is a political, policy and practice willingness to support an EpiCrim approach to the***

prevention of and response to sexual abuse but that there needs to be better streamlined, and more evidence-based multi-agency working to allow political cover in doing so.

Section Two: Prevention

Section two of the book examines some of the challenges facing sexual abuse prevention (primary and secondary prevention across the individual, interpersonal, community and societal levels) in the EpiCrim model. **Addis, Rees, Johnson, Legg, and Brennan** (Chapter 5) discuss the challenges and opportunities for sexual abuse, especially CSA, prevention in the online world arguing that social media platforms need to do more to safeguard children and young people, while placing this debate within the context of a shifting policy (i.e. online harms bill and the development of Artificial Intelligence) and practice (i.e. working with social media companies, internet providers, and criminal justice organisations). The chapter argues that the shifting perception of the role of online and offline worlds in the lives of children and young people should give us a point to pause and reflect, rather than rush to poorly developed policy and practice. This is expanded upon in the next two chapters by **Rees and Bovill** (Chapter 6) as well as **Meyrick** (Chapter 7) who argue that there needs to be better understandings of the early signs, risks and opportunities to intervene to prevent sexual abuse by professionals. With Rees and Bovill arguing that frontline staff training, in this instance police officers, needs to continue its development of an adaptable and evidence-based understanding of the reality of violence against women and girls, with Merrick building on this to state that all frontline staff need to better understand how to facilitate, manage and respond to sexual abuse disclosures. These two chapters highlight the need for better staff development and the need for an informed workforce, which ties with the **Addis et al.** chapter in which they argue that there is a social responsibility for understanding sexual abuse prevention that needs to be ingrained in all organisations and communities in society, so that individuals can intervene where appropriate.

The main finding from section two is that th***e prevention of sexual abuse is possible, but it needs an individual and interpersonal response that is only possible by upskilling communities and putting prevention at the heart for their activities through changing the over-arching social norms around it. Additionally, the section argues that sexual abuse prevention, although structurally different, is an important in the online world as it is in the offline one.***

Section Three: Treatment and Rehabilitation

Section three of the book examines some of the challenges facing the treatment and rehabilitation of men convicted of a sexual offence (tertiary prevention across the individual, interpersonal, community, and societal levels) in the EpiCrim model. This section focuses on research, policy and practice linked to trauma informed care with people convicted of a sexual offence, which is important as there is a lot of research evidence from America, Canada, Australia, and New Zealand for example, but there is less from the UK. Pawson, **Senker, & Eason** (Chapter 8) discuss the challenges and opportunities for developing an evidence base in trauma informed practice for men convicted of a sexual offence. They argue that there needs to be a policy and practice shift in understanding that the past traumas of men convicted of a sexual offence can be a core part of their offending trajectory, and therefore their rehabilitation and social integration. In the chapter, Senker et al. argue that to have functional EpiCrim approach to release prevention there needs to be a coherent and fit for purpose trauma informed system in place. This approach is reinforced and built on by **Prescott** (Chapter 9) as well as **Jones and Ackerman** (Chapter 10) who discuss the clinical, rehabilitative and professional skills needed to facilitate trauma informed interventions. Prescott talks about this in an individual and interpersonal level through one-on-one therapy and Ackerman and Jones at the interpersonal and community levels through their work in therapeutic communities. Both chapters reinforce the system-wide changes, and the ideological shift needed towards a trauma informed approach that is necessary to ensure that an EpiCrim approach is viable. This section is completed with a chapter from **Eason** (Chapter 10) on the importance of providing trauma informed care and support for professionals who work with people, particularly men, who have committed sexual abuse. In the chapter, Eason argues that professional safeguarding and care is important for preventing burn out in staff as well for guaranteeing the quality of care that service users receive. Trauma informed practice is essential in therapeutic interventions and work to support community safety, risk management and desistance from offending.

The main finding from section three was that ***good therapeutic interventions, rehabilitation and community re-entry is based on trauma informed practice that support service users and staff equally. This means that individual, interpersonal and community-based trauma informed responses help to protect communities and societies from future sexual harm from individuals.***

Section Four: Community Integration, Harm Reduction and Desistence

Section four of the book examines some of the challenges facing the community and societal integration of men convicted of a sexual offence (quaternary prevention across the individual, interpersonal, community and societal levels) in the EpiCrim model. Quaternary prevention is a relatively new concept, and therefore the most underdeveloped prevention stage in respect to sexual abuse (McCartan & Kemshall, 2023). In this context, quaternary prevention forces community integration, desistance and harm reduction. The two chapters in his section speak to the importance of integration, community acceptance, and "moving on" in the lives of people with a conviction for a sexual offence. **Gavin, Cawley, Kewley, Burke, Wager and Porter** (Chapter 12) discuss the role of restorative justice in cases of sexual abuse, often a controversial practice in the eyes of criminal justice and some victim's organisations, and how it can help in the desistance and integration process. The chapter emphases the roles of understanding, compassion, communication and the continuance of a therapeutic process in the community. This is built on by **Porter and Merdian** (Chapter 13) who discuss the challenges of employment for people, particularly men, convicted of a sexual offence and how more work needs to be done in this area. The chapter argues that employment and meaningful work is import in the integration and risk management process, but to achieve the employer myths need to be challenged and communities as well as society need to buy into the rehabilitee aspect of prison and probation.

The main finding from section four is that **harm reduction and social inclusion is possible with men convicted of a sexual offence but only through changing social ideas about what is good practice and to effectively risk manage the process. Community and societal change are need to successfully achieve harm reduction and desistence from sexual offending at the individual and interpersonal levels.**

Overall Conclusion

The book shows that the EpiCrim approach is a viable framework for understanding how we respond to and prevent sexual abuse across the socio-ecological model and gives credence to the policy and practice of governments, organisations and practices that already do this. The book highlights that we need to think about sexual abuse in all aspects of sexual abuse prevention (primary, secondary, tertiary, and quaternary) across all socio-ecological levels (individual, interpersonal, community, and societal) and all forms of sexual abuse. Understanding and responding to sexual abuse in a public health frame means thinking as much about the individual as the context in which the harm occurs which reflects the bio-psycho-social model and calls for us to be more innovate in how we approach it. Which means that to best understand how to prevent and respond to sexual abuse we need to focus equally at every stage of the socio-ecological model (*individual, interpersonal, community, and societal*) developing appropriate interventions that reflect the nuances of a range of sexual abuse (*i.e. rape, child sexual abuse, harmful sexual behaviour in children and young people, online sexual abuse, and contact sexual abuse*) and the diversity of the individuals and populations involved in them (*i.e. focusing on age, gender, mental health, neurodiversity, race, culture, and community*) (see Fig. 14.1).

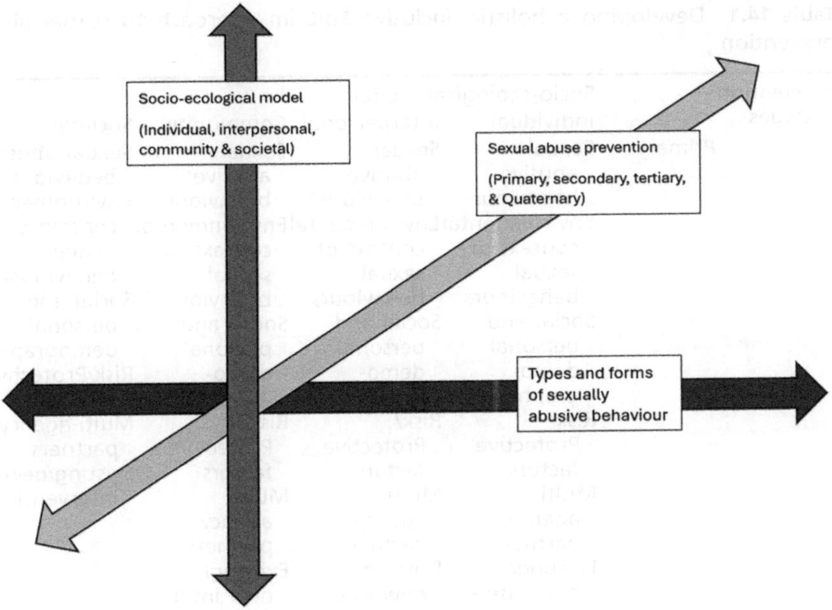

Fig. 14.1 The intersection of EpiCrim components in the prevention of sexual abuse

The book has highlighted that there needs to be a rounded and grounded socio-cultural and socio-political conversation about the reality of sexual abuse, with a system-wide approach being the only real way to tackle it (see Table 14.1).

However, this is complicated and will not happen easily, which is why a top down and bottom-up approach is necessary (McCartan, 2022) which means changing individuals and communities understanding on sexual abuse while developing and implementing regional and national government policies (Fig. 14.2).

The book has highlighted that the EpiCrim approach works across a range of sexually abusive behaviours and populations (i.e. CSA, HSB-CYP, adult on adult sexual abuse, online sexual abuse, and misogyny) and opens up the model to be used in new as well as innovative ways with different populations, for instance, children and young people with autism (Russell et al., 2025; Russell et al., in press).

Table 14.1 Developing a holistic, inclusive EpiCrim approach to sexual abuse prevention

Prevention stages		Socio-ecological model			
		Individual	Interpersonal	Community	Societal
	Primary	Sexual abusive behaviour Environmental context of sexual behaviours Social and personal demographics Risk/Protective factors Multi-agency partners Existing/new interventions	Sexual abusive behaviour Environmental context of sexual behaviours Social and personal demographics Risk/Protective factors Multi-agency partners Existing/new interventions	Sexual abusive behaviour Environmental context of sexual behaviours Social and personal demographics Risk/Protective factors Multi-agency partners Existing/new interventions	Sexual abusive behaviour Environmental context of sexual behaviours Social and personal demographics Risk/Protective factors Multi-agency partners Existing/new interventions
	Secondary	Sexual abusive behaviour Environmental context of sexual behaviours Social and personal demographics Risk/Protective factors Multi-agency partners Existing/new interventions	Sexual abusive behaviour Environmental context of sexual behaviours Social and personal demographics Risk/Protective factors Multi-agency partners Existing/new interventions	Sexual abusive behaviour Environmental context of sexual behaviours Social and personal demographics Risk/Protective factors Multi-agency partners Existing/new interventions	Sexual abusive behaviour Environmental context of sexual behaviours Social and personal demographics Risk/Protective factors Multi-agency partners Existing/new interventions

(continued)

Table 14.1 (continued)

Tertiary	Sexual abusive behaviour Environmental context of sexual behaviours Social and personal demo-graphics Risk/Protective factors Multi-agency partners Existing/new inter-ventions	Sexual abusive behaviour Environmental context of sexual behaviours Social and personal demo-graphics Risk/Protective factors Multi-agency partners Existing/new inter-ventions	Sexual abusive behaviour Environmental context of sexual behaviours Social and personal demo-graphics Risk/Protective factors Multi-agency partners Existing/new inter-ventions	Sexual abusive behaviour Environmental context of sexual behaviours Social and personal demographics Risk/Protective factors Multi-agency partners Existing/new interventions
Quaternary	Sexual abusive behaviour Environmental context of sexual behaviours Social and personal demo-graphics Risk/Protective factors Multi-agency partners Existing/new inter-ventions	Sexual abusive behaviour Environmental context of sexual behaviours Social and personal demo-graphics Risk/Protective factors Multi-agency partners Existing/new inter-ventions	Sexual abusive behaviour Environmental context of sexual behaviours Social and personal demo-graphics Risk/Protective factors Multi-agency partners Existing/new inter-ventions	Sexual abusive behaviour Environmental context of sexual behaviours Social and personal demographics Risk/Protective factors Multi-agency partners Existing/new interventions

Recommendations and Future Directions

The book enforces that an EpiCrim approach is a relevant way of understanding preventing and responding to sex abuse, therefore it is important to consider how we can use this approach most effectively

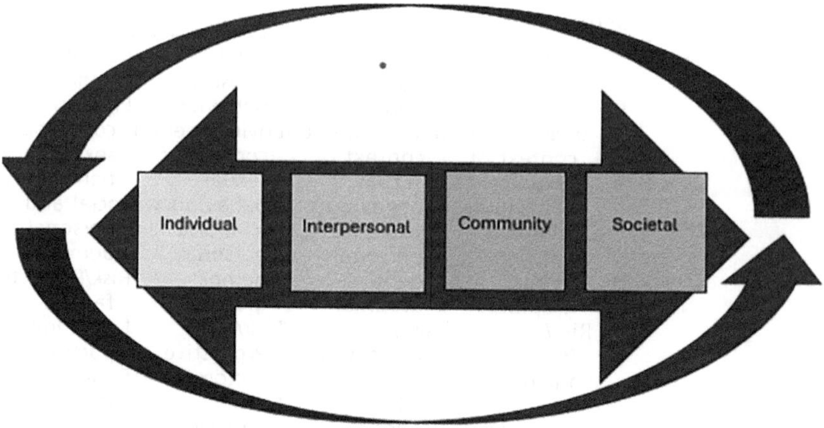

Fig. 14.2 The interrelationship between the socio-ecological model and inclusive sexual abuse prevention

to influence policy, practice and research. Based on the contents of this book, the following recommendations for future policy, practice, and research flow.

1. The EpiCrim framework ties health, public health, social work, social care and criminal justice together in a cohesive way to understand all forms of sexual abuse across the socio-ecology model and therefore should be used to develop, roll out and evaluate all forms of prevention.
2. Current research and evidence indicate that more work needs to be done in framing sexual abuse prevention at the community and society level, as most of the work that has been done to date is at the individual and interpersonal level. If communities are where sexual abuse occurs and if they are shaped and ascertain individual as well as societal view on the issue, then they are the lynchpin for better understanding to respond and prevent it.
3. Currently, there is a need to develop more robust evaluation frameworks and key performance indicators for EpiCrim, especially the secondary and quaternary prevention levels across all stages of the socio-ecological model. Therefore, academics, policy makers, and

practitioners should come together to develop, implement and test them.

4. There is the need to develop local, national and transnationally policies and practices that emphasise the importance of an EpiCrim approach. While there are policies at a transnational level through organisations like the United Nations, European Union and World Health Organisation, they are more specifically the national level. This is problematic as it means that transnationally policies are never truly operationalised as there is no national or local infrastructure.
5. EpiCrim approaches to sexual abuse responses and prevention emphasise a multi-agency approach, but this needs more work and more strategic development. In addition, it's important to think about how we engage in primary and secondary prevention, across the socio-ecological model, in a multi-agency way. How can first time or early-stage prevention of sexual abuse be framed, and rolled out, in the same fashion as relapse prevention? We would propose that an array of different government agencies and departments can be utilised to work collectively to respond to sexual abuse in a holistic way.
6. The EpiCrim approach encourages a harm reduction framework through discussion of quaternary prevention, and this needs to be better conceptualised in criminal justice, especially in cases of sexual abuse. The book emphasises the importance of integration and desistence through inclusion, redemption, treatment and employability all of which need to better develop and implemented.
7. That the term violence against women and girls is too limiting given the nature and scale of sexual abuse committed against boys, therefore the term violence against women and children should be used as it's more inclusive.
8. An EpiCrim approach emphasises the importance of a holistic, life-course trauma informed approach to understanding offending behaviour. This means that therapeutic, mental health, and wellbeing interventions for people convicted of a sexual offence needs to take account of their adverse life experiences and enable them to be supported in their recovery from any victimisation that they

many have suffered. Which is a challenging socio-political issue, but one that needs to be addressed.

9. An EpiCrim approach emphasises the importance of better funded and broader victim support services. Better and more timely victim services may lead to a reduction in future sexual abuse by individuals who sexually offend who have experienced their own with adverse childhood and life experiences.
10. A trauma informed approach needs to operate in a trauma informed system, which means better support for staff both in terms of their previous trauma, ongoing first-hand trauma as well as vicarious trauma linked to their roles. Working within the field of sexual abuse is challenging and can be triggering for people, therefore it is the responsibility of their employer and the state to support them.

The recommendations that have emerged from the book emphasise that sexual abuse is complex and nuanced but is preventable. If we see sexual abuse as a social issue that impacts individuals through their relationships with each other and the multiple communities that they are a member of, we can proactively work to reduce it. An EpiCrim approach allows us to view sexual abuse in a rounded and grounded light, which enables us to develop bespoke and a fit for purpose response.

References

Brown, J. (2017). *Public health, prevention and risk management*. In K. Mccartan & H. Kemshall (Eds.), *Contemporary sex offender risk management, Volume I: Perceptions*. Palgrave MacMillan.

ECPAT International. (2024). *Scoping review of international approaches to child sexual abuse and exploitation prevention interventions by law enforcement*. ECPAT International.

King-Hill, S. (2022). *Child sexual abuse review: Listening to children and young people is crucial.* The conversation. Retrieved from https://theconversation.com/child-sexual-abuse-review-listening-to-children-and-young-people-is-crucial-193356

McCartan, K. F. (2022). Translating the sexual abuse evidence base into effective policy and practice. In K. Uzieblo, W. Smid, & K. F. McCartan (Eds.), *At the crossroads: Future directions in sex offender treatment and management*. Palgrave MacMillan.

McCartan, K., & Kemshall, H. (2020). The potential role of recovery capital in stopping sexual offending: Lessons from circles of support and accountability to enrich practice. *Irish Probation Journal, 17*, 87–106. http://www.probation.ie/EN/PB/0/1B01C0821143FED68025862C005298DC/$File/Kieran%20McCartan%20and%20Hazel%20Kemshall.pdf

Russell, D., McCartan, K., & King-Hill, S. (2025). *Multi-systemic responses and understanding to the prevention and intervention of harmful sexual behaviour in autistic children and young people*. Association for the Treatment and Prevention of Sexual Abuse blog. Retrieved from https://blog.atsa.com/

Russell, D., King-Hill, S., Allardyce, S., & Allely, C. (in press). *Harmful sexual behaviour and autism. Working with children and young people*. Jessica Kingsley.

9783031936333